THE BIOLOGY AND PREVENTION OF AERODIGESTIVE TRACT CANCERS

ADVANCES IN EXPERIMENTAL MEDICINE AND BIOLOGY

THE BIOLOGY AND PREVENTION OF AERODIGESTIVE TRACT CANCERS

Edited by

Guy R. Newell and Waun Ki Hong

The University of Texas M. D. Anderson Cancer Center
Houston, Texas

SPRINGER SCIENCE+BUSINESS MEDIA, LLC

Library of Congress Cataloging-in-Publication Data

The Biology and prevention of aerodigestive tract cancers / edited by
  Guy R. Newell and Waun Ki. Hong.
      p.   cm. -- (Advances in experimental medicine and biology ; v.
  320)
    "Proceedings of a conference ... held February 21-23, 1991 in
  Houston, Texas"--T.p. verso.
    Published for the University of Texas M.D. Anderson Cancer Center,
  Houston, Texas"--T.p. verso.
    Includes bibliographical references and index.
    ISBN 978-1-4613-6536-5   ISBN 978-1-4615-3468-6 (eBook)
    DOI 10.1007/978-1-4615-3468-6
    1. Mouth--Cancer--Etiology--Congresses. 2. Mouth--Cancer-
  -Chemoprevention--Congresses. 3. Throat--Cancer--Etiology-
  -Congresses. 4. Throat--Cancer--Chemoprevention--Congresses.
  I. Newell, Guy R. II. Hong, Waun Ki. III. University of Texas M.D.
  Anderson Cancer Center. IV. Series.
    [DNLM: 1. Head and Neck Neoplasms--congresses.   W1 AD559 v.320 /
  WE 707 B615]
  RC280.B6B56 1992
  DNLM/DLC
  for Library of Congress   92-21811
                                                                 CIP

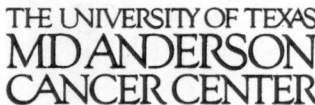

THE UNIVERSITY OF TEXAS
MD ANDERSON
CANCER CENTER

Golden Jubilee
SHINING
PAST
BRILLIANT
FUTURE
1941-1991

Published for
The University of Texas M. D. Anderson Cancer Center, Houston, Texas,
by Plenum Publishing Corporation, New York

Proceedings of a conference on The Biology and Prevention of
Aerodigestive Tract Cancers, held February 21-23, 1991, in Houston, Texas

ISBN 978-1-4613-6536-5

© 1992 Springer Science+Business Media New York
Originally published by Plenum Press, New York in 1992

PREFACE

The papers contained in this volume were presented at the Golden Jubilee Cancer Prevention Conference, "The Biology and Prevention of Aerodigestive Tract Cancers," sponsored by The University of Texas M. D. Anderson Cancer Center in Houston, Texas, February 21–23, 1991. The purpose of the conference was to further the understanding of the biology, epidemiology, and prevention of aerodigestive tract cancers. Advances in understanding the biology of aerodigestive tract cancers have led to successful early chemoprevention trials. Chemopreventive agents in current use are capable of reversing premalignant lesions, as well as reducing the number of second primary cancers of the head and neck. These trials hold the promise that effective prevention methods for these cancers will be forthcoming in the foreseeable future. Carcinogenic exposures appear to affect the entire epithelial lining of the upper aerodigestive tract, a phenomena described as "field cancerization." This process contributes to the development of both synchronous and metachronous aerodigestive tract cancers. It also provides a sound rationale for the chemoprevention of these cancers. Animal models are important for identifying the critical components of field cancerization and for testing potentially new chemopreventive agents and regimens. The hamster lung carcinogenesis model and the hamster cheek model are discussed.

Aerodigestive tract cancers account for about 20% of newly diagnosed invasive cancers. Cigarette smoking and alcohol consumption are the most important risk factors for these cancers. Smokeless tobacco is clearly associated with the development of oral leukoplakia, which is a premalignant lesion. Individuals who use smokeless tobacco tend not to be cigarette smokers. Both vitamin A and β-carotene intake have been associated with a decrease in lung cancer risk. Although alcohol is known to be synergistic with tobacco smoke, data are presented that suggest alcohol is not only an independent risk factor but should also be considered a cocarcinogen acting through the interference with DNA repair. Intermediate biomarkers, such as bleomycin-induced chromosome breaks in cultured lymphocytes, will be important in determining the interaction between genetic factors and environmental exposures. Biomarkers will also be useful in assessing individual sensitivity for the development of both initial and subsequent cancers in these sites.

Several chapters describe some molecular aspects of field cancerization, some of which include oncogene abnormalities, retinoic acid receptors, and retinoid-responsive genes. These molecular events provide mechanisms through which retinoid chemoprevention may be accomplished. Oncogene abnormalities now associated with lung cancer may also predispose to the development of other aerodigestive tract cancers.

Detailed descriptions of ongoing chemoprevention trials are presented. These include issues of both design and implementation, as well as of several ongoing clinical trials. Differences between chemoprevention trials and clinical trials are stressed, emphasizing long-term adherence and maintenance of sufficient subjects to provide enough statistical power to demonstrate an intervention effect. Development of reliable intermediate end points would greatly improve the efficiency of these trials. Trials performed at M. D. Anderson Cancer

Center include studies of oral leukoplakia and second primary tumors of the head and neck. Chemoprevention trials using both synthetic retinoids, namely 13-*cis*–retinoic acid and natural agents, retinol and β-carotene, are reviewed.

In summary, this volume presents an update on the biology, epidemiology, and prevention of aerodigestive tract cancers. The biology emphasizes the concept of field cancerization and its quantitation by the use of new intermediate biomarkers. The prevention emphasizes recent successes in the chemoprevention of oral leukoplakia and second primary cancers of the head and neck. These successes serve as excellent models for the future chemoprevention of these important cancer sites.

Guy R. Newell
Waun Ki Hong

ACKNOWLEDGMENTS

Financial support was generously provided by grant no. 1R13-CA54775-01 from the National Cancer Institute, National Institutes of Health and from the Physician Oncology Education Program, Texas Cancer Council.

We gratefully acknowledge the expert editorial support of Diane F. Bush, managing editor, who was assisted by Gayle Nesom, Jude Richard, Edith K. Wilson, and Cynthia Albers of the Department of Scientific Publications, The University of Texas M. D. Anderson Cancer Center, Houston, Texas.

CONTENTS

The Etiology and Prevention of Aerodigestive Tract Cancers

David Schottenfeld

Department of Epidemiology
University of Michigan
School of Public Health
Ann Arbor, Michigan

INTRODUCTION

In the United States, the currently estimated number of deaths owing to upper digestive (oral cavity, pharynx, and esophagus) and respiratory (larynx and lung) tract cancers represents almost 40% of the overall cancer mortality rate in males and 23% in females. Of the approximately 1,040,000 incidences of cancers in men and women estimated for 1990 in the United States, 20% have been diagnosed in the aerodigestive tract (Table 1) (1). Aerodigestive tract cancer incidence rates appear more commonly in males throughout the world, where the male:female incidence ratios may vary between 2 and 6, and, within most geographic areas, vary inversely with socioeconomic status. In North America and Western Europe, the major risk factors for aerodigestive tract squamous cell carcinomas (SCCs) are alcohol and tobacco. Approximately 140,000 deaths in the United States each year, owing to upper digestive and respiratory tract cancers, can be attributed to cigarette smoking and alcohol consumption.

DEMOGRAPHIC PATTERNS

Oral Cavity and Pharynx

Age-adjusted oral and pharyngeal cancer mortality in the United States in 1987 was 2.8 times higher in males (5.6×10^{-5}) than in females (2.0×10^{-5}), and 1.7 times higher in blacks (5.7×10^{-5}) than in whites (3.4×10^{-5}). The age-specific death rates increased exponentially with increasing age in white males and females, whereas in blacks, the rates appeared to peak at ages 55–64 years, and then remained at the same level in the older age groups (Figure 1). Age-adjusted mortality rates in the past 15 years declined by 20% in whites and increased by 8% in blacks. Age-adjusted incidence rates during the same period declined minimally (about 2%) in the white males and females, increased by 34% in the black males, and was essentially unchanged, apart from sampling fluctuations, in the black females (Figure 2) (2).

In the United States, the most common site among black males is the pharynx, whereas among white males, it is the oral cavity. The most frequently diagnosed subsites in the oral cavity are the tongue and gum (Table 2). Moore and Catlin (3) described a high-risk horseshoe-

The Biology and Prevention of Aerodigestive Tract Cancers
Edited by G.R.Newell and W.K. Hong, Plenum Press, New York, 1992

1

Table 1. Estimated New Cancer Cases and Deaths for 1990, United States

	Incidences				Deaths			
	Males	(%)	Females	(%)	Males	(%)	Females	(%)
All sites	520,000	(100.0)	520,000	(100.0)	270,000	(100.0)	240,000	(100.0)
Oral cavity and pharynx	20,400	(3.9)	10,100	(1.9)	5,575	(2.1)	2,775	(1.2)
Esophagus	7,400	(1.4)	3,200	(0.6)	7,000	(2.6)	2,500	(1.0)
Larynx	10,000	(1.9)	2,300	(0.4)	3,000	(1.1)	750	(0.3)
Lung	102,000	(19.6)	55,000	(10.6)	92,000	(34.1)	50,000	(20.8)
Subtotal[a]	139,800	(26.8)	70,600	(13.5)	107,575	(39.9)	56,025	(23.3)

[a]Upper digestive tract and respiratory tract.
Source: *1990 Cancer Facts and Figures*, American Cancer Society. Incidence estimates are based on rates from the NCI SEER Program, 1984–1986.

shaped mucosal region that extends backward from the anterior floor of the mouth, over both lingual-alveolar sulci and lateral margins of the anterior two thirds of the tongue, and then finally reaches the anterior tonsillar pillar and retromolar trigone area.

The age-adjusted incidence of oral and pharyngeal cancers varies more than 20-fold throughout the world. The highest incidence among males is reported in France, with annual rates exceeding 40 per 100,000 in the east-central part of the country along the German border (Bas-Rhin) and on the Brittany coast (Calvados). The highest incidence among females is reported in India (Table 3) (4). Although in most parts of the world, oral cancer occurs more frequently in males, higher rates for females are reported in the Phillipines, in Singapore and Bangalore among Indians, and in Iceland. In India and other parts of Central Asia, a major risk factor for oral cancer is tobacco, which can be chewed as a betel quid or smoked.

Esophagus

One of the most intriguing features of esophageal cancer is its geographic variability. The pattern around the world resembles a mosaic of contrasting incidence rates and sex ratios. The mosaic incidence pattern is not restricted to natural geographic boundaries, but rather appears to reflect a complex of environmental factors that are intimately correlated with sociocultural and ethnic characteristics. In most parts of the world, incidence rates per 100,000 are around

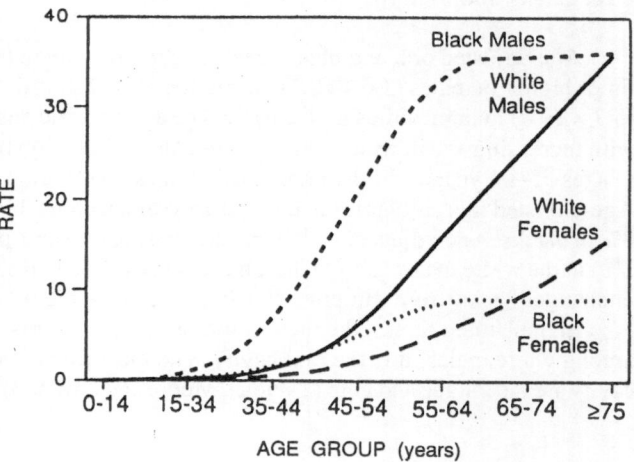

Figure 1. Age-specific death rates per 100,000 from oral cavity and pharyngeal cancer, white and black males and females (United States, 1987).

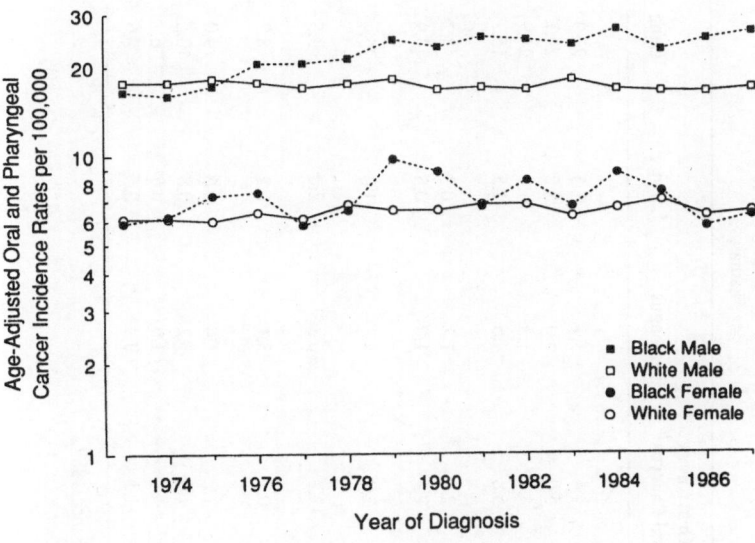

Figure 2. Age-adjusted oral and pharyngeal cancer incidence rates per 100,000, by sex and race (U.S. SEER Program, 1973–1987).

2.5 to 5.0 for males and 1.5 to 2.5 for females, but they may exceed 100.0 in areas of Asia to the north and east of the Caspian Sea. In high-incidence areas such as India, the Transkei (southern Africa), and the Gonbad region in northern Iran, the incidence in females approaches or exceeds that in males. In the northwestern part of Iran, the actuarial risk of developing esophageal cancer before age 65 is approximately one in six. Over 60% of the annual esophageal cancer deaths in the world are reported in China, where it is the second most common cancer after stomach cancer. The mortality rates in high-risk areas in northern China exceed 100 per 100,000, and include the provinces of Honan, Hopei, Shansi, and Kwangtung (5).

In the United States, the average annual age-adjusted incidence rate per 100,000 for esophageal cancer is 5.3 in white males and 1.7 in white females; the rate in black males is 19.4 and in black females, 5.0. The relative percentage increase in age-adjusted incidence during the period from 1973–1974 to 1986–1987 was 9.5% in white males and 21.2% in black males. In addition to the blacks in the United States, elevated incidence rates occur in Hawaiians and

Table 2. Average Annual Age-adjusted[a] Mortality Rates per 100,000, Site-Specific Within Aerodigestive Tract, United States, 1983–1987

Site	Total	Males	Females
Oral cavity and pharynx	2.9	4.5	1.7
Lip	0.0	0.1	0.0
Tongue	0.7	1.0	0.4
Salivary gland	0.2	0.3	0.1
Floor of mouth	0.1	0.2	0.1
Gum and other parts of mouth	0.5	0.7	0.3
Nasopharynx	0.2	0.3	0.1
Tonsil	0.2	0.3	0.1
Oropharynx	0.2	0.3	0.1
Hypopharynx	0.2	0.4	0.1
Esophagus	2.8	4.8	1.2
Lung and bronchus	45.8	72.2	26.6
Larynx	1.3	2.4	0.4
Nose, nasal cavity, and middle ear	0.5	0.8	0.3

[a]1970 U.S. standard population.

Table 3. Age-standardized Incidence Rate per 100,000: Cancers of Oral Cavity and Pharynx (ICD-9:141,143–146,148,149), Esophagus (ICD-9:150), Larynx (ICD-9:161), and Lung (ICD-9:162) for Selected Populations, Males and Females, 1980[a]

Country/City	Race/Ethnicity	Males				Females			
		Oral Cavity and Pharynx[b]	Esophagus	Larynx	Lung	Oral Cavity and Pharynx[b]	Esophagus	Larynx	Lung
United States									
Detroit, MI	Whites	11.2	4.4	8.4	75.5	4.4	1.1	1.5	27.9
	Blacks	18.9	16.9	10.6	102.3	5.0	5.0	2.2	29.7
Atlanta, GA	Whites	10.5	4.0	7.5	77.1	4.6	1.3	1.4	24.9
	Blacks	20.2	17.1	11.5	94.6	5.8	4.6	1.5	15.2
France									
Calvados		44.2	29.9	10.3	43.6	2.6	1.2	0.3	3.2
Bas-Rhin		46.5	16.7	12.4	60.2	2.5	1.0	0.5	3.9
United Kingdom, Scotland		4.5	8.0	4.6	91.1	2.2	4.2	1.0	26.4
Bombay, India		32.7	14.7	10.0	15.7	12.7	10.3	2.0	3.5
Miyagi, Japan		2.2	13.3	2.2	29.6	0.7	3.1	0.2	8.7
Israel	All Jews (Total)	2.1	1.9	5.5	27.9	1.2	1.4	0.6	9.0
	Jews (European/American)	1.5	1.9	5.1	29.9	1.0	1.2	0.8	10.6
	Jews (African/Asian)	2.7	35.8	6.1	31.5	1.1	1.6	0.6	6.1
	Non-Jews	2.8	1.0	4.9	23.4	1.3	0.9	0.5	3.6

[a]Source: Modified from Cancer Incidence in Five Continents, vol. V. International Agency for Research on Cancer, Lyon, France, 1987.
[b]Oral cavity and pharynx excludes lip, salivary gland, and nasopharynx.

Alaskan Eskimos and Aleuts, in contrast to the low risks exhibited by Hispanics (New Mexico) and American Indians (Figure 3). The incidence among Puerto Rican males is similar to that in U.S. black males.

During 1973–1987, the reported incidence of SCC of the esophagus in U.S. white and black men and women was relatively stable. However, adenocarcinoma of the esophagus increased more than 100% in white and black men, and by about 50% in white women. The black:white age-adjusted incidence ratio in men was 5.6 for SCC and 0.3 for adenocarcinoma. A similar pattern was exhibited in the women. By 1987, adenocarcinoma accounted for 34% of all esophageal cancers in white men, 12% in white women, 3% in black men, and 1% in black women. The very high male:female ratio, higher incidence among whites, and significantly increasing incidence during the past two decades associated with adenocarcinoma of the esophagus was also reported for adenocarcinoma of the gastric cardia (6). At least 80% of the adenocarcinomas appeared in the lower third of the esophagus, frequently in conjunction with Barrett's columnar metaplasia, which was more common in men than in women. and in whites than in blacks. The histogenesis of the columnar epithelial metaplasia was believed to be secondary to chronic inflammatory injury, as a result of severe gastroesophageal reflux, cytotoxic chemotherapy, or other chemical agents that may cause mucosal ulcerations (7). The specific epidemiologic determinants of adenocarcinoma of the esophagus, when distinguished from SCC, have not been established; in particular, the potential role of alcohol and tobacco would not have adequately explained the contrasting demographic patterns described for the two cell types of carcinoma.

Larynx

The average annual incidence rate per 100,000 for laryngeal cancer in the United States is 2.3 for glottic and 1.3 for supraglottic subsites. The male:female incidence ratio is 3.5 for supraglottic and 9.5 for glottic carcinomas (8). By way of comparison, the male:female incidence ratio for lung cancer is currently 2–3:1 in U.S. whites and blacks, respectively. The age-adjusted incidence rate per 100,000 for total laryngeal cancer is 12.7 in black males, 8.4 in white males, 2.6 in black females, and 1.6 in white females. The relative percentage change in age-adjusted incidence during this period from 1973–1974 to 1986–1987 was +3.7% in white males and +19.7% in black males. For lung cancer, during a comparable period encompassed by the Surveillance, Epidemiology and End Results (SEER) Program (National Institutes of Health), the relative percentage change in age-adjusted incidence was +12% in white males and +21% in black males (9).

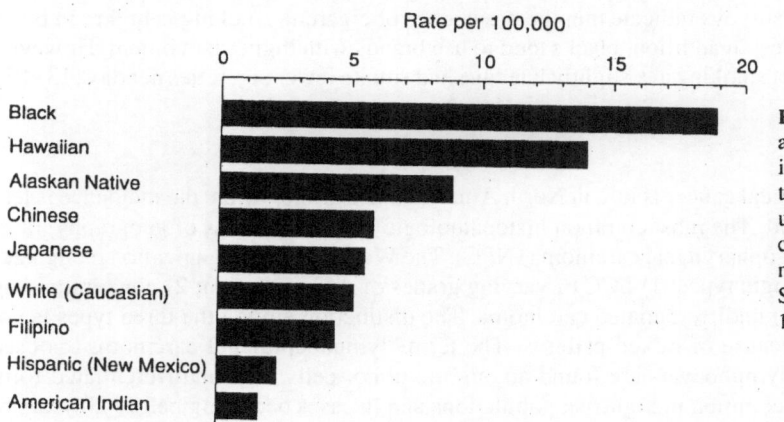

Rate per 100,000

Figure 3. Average annual age-adjusted incidence rates (i.e., to the 1970 U.S. population) per 100,000, cancer of esophagus, males by race (U.S. SEER Program, 1977–1983).

The incidence of cancer of the larynx varies worldwide; it is generally predominant in males, and the rates in females are relatively uniform and at a level below 1.5 per 100,000. The magnitude of laryngeal cancer may not vary in any constant or predictable relationship to the incidence of lung cancer in the same population. In the United Kingdom, laryngeal cancer incidence is relatively low, and lung cancer incidence is quite high. In the Mediterranean countries, India and Central Asia, the increased incidence rates of laryngeal cancer are not, in general, associated with high lung cancer incidence rates, but are significantly correlated with increased oral, pharyngeal, and esophageal cancer incidences. As noted by McMichael (10), laryngeal cancer mortality rates reported in industrialized nations are more significantly correlated with per capita alcohol consumption than with tobacco consumption.

Lung and Bronchus

Lung cancer is the leading cause of cancer mortality in the United States. From 1980 to 1987, the age-adjusted lung cancer mortality rate per 100,000 increased from 46.2 to 52.1. In 1987, the lung cancer mortality rate in women (28.2) exceeded that of breast cancer (27.1). Among U.S. black males, lung cancer mortality is the second leading cause of death, ranking below coronary heart disease. The risk of dying of lung cancer for black males is at least 1.5 times higher than that for white males; there is no significant difference in risk between white and black females. The excess mortality from lung cancer among black males compared with white males is greatest for the age interval, 35–64 years.

The age-adjusted lung cancer incidence in males increased nearly 1% per year between 1973 and 1982; since 1983, there has been a lesser rate of increase of +0.6% per year. In white and black females, lung cancer incidence, since 1973, has increased 5.4% per year.

Among males, the maximum exposure to tobacco, which accounts for approximately 85% of incident lung cancer cases, was experienced by those born between 1910 and 1920, whereas among women, the peak in smoking prevalence was experienced by those born between 1930 and 1940. Declining lung cancer mortality in men was first manifested in those born after 1935; in women, lung cancer mortality is currently declining in the subgroups younger than 50 years of age, or in those born after 1940. Smoking prevalence has decreased among adult men and women, from 40% in 1965 to 29% in 1987 (11,12).

Compared with women, men generally begin to smoke cigarettes at an earlier age, smoke more cigarettes per day and for a longer duration, inhale more deeply, and consume cigarettes with higher tar content. The Federal Trade Commission estimated that the current average sales-weighted tar content of cigarettes manufactured in the United States is about 12–13 mg of tar per cigarette, compared with nearly 40 mg in the early 1950s. In the United States, it has been estimated that the cumulative exposure to tobacco in women has been only 40% of that in men. National surveys indicate that the prevalence of cigarette smoking is higher in black than in white males; in addition, blacks tend to use brands with higher tar content. However, blacks tend to start smoking at a slightly later age and smoke fewer cigarettes per day (13–15).

Nasopharynx

Nasopharyngeal cancer is rare in North America and Europe, where the incidence is less than 1 per 100,000. The most common histopathologic form, regardless of geography, race, or ethnicity, is nasopharyngeal carcinoma (NPC). The World Health Organization recognizes three histopathologic types: 1) SCC of varying grades of differentiation; 2) nonkeratinizing carcinoma; and 3) undifferentiated carcinoma. The distinction among the three types is not often possible because of mixed patterns. The term "lymphoepithelial carcinoma" is used when numerous lymphocytes are found among the tumor cells. The undifferentiated form tends to be more common in high-risk populations and in cases occurring before 20 years of age.

In contrast to the race-specific incidence pattern described in Figure 4 for lung cancer in the United States, where risks are high in blacks and Hawaiians, intermediate in Chinese and Japanese, and low in Filipinos and Hispanics (New Mexico), the pattern for NPC reveals markedly elevated incidences in the Chinese; intermediate in Filipinos; and low in the Hispanics, blacks, and Japanese (Figure 5). While NPC is rare in Japan, it is common in specific regions of China and Southeast Asia. The Chinese from the southern provinces of Canton, Kwangsi, and Fukien are at significantly higher risk than those from the northern provinces of Peking, Tientsin, and Shanghai. The epidemiologic features of NPC are summarized in Table 4 (16).

There is mounting seroepidemiologic and molecular biologic evidence that the Epstein-Barr virus (EBV) is an etiologic agent in NPC (17,18). EBV genomes that are transcriptionally active have been detected in the tumor tissue from biopsy specimens all over the world. The increased risk of NPC in genetically distinct subpopulations of Chinese origin has suggested that genetic susceptibility is necessary for tumor induction. Chinese patients with NPC demonstrate an increase in the frequency of the first locus human leukocyte antigen (HLA), A2, and the second locus antigen, BW46. However, there is little indication that there is a common universal HLA system complex that correlates consistently with NPC, but conceivably there may be other linkages with genes controlling susceptibility and pathogenesis. The evidence available does not yet support the conclusion that EBV alone is both the necessary and the sufficient cause of NPC in high- and low-risk populations.

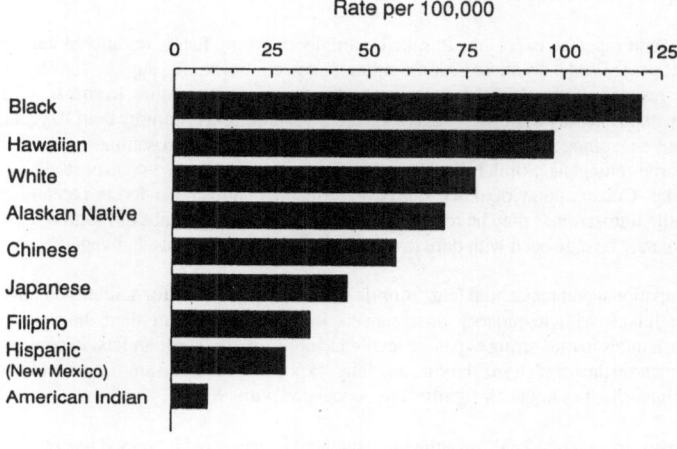

Figure 4. Average annual age-adjusted incidence rates (i.e., to the 1970 U.S. population) per 100,000, cancer of lung and bronchus, males by race (U.S. SEER Program, 1977–1983).

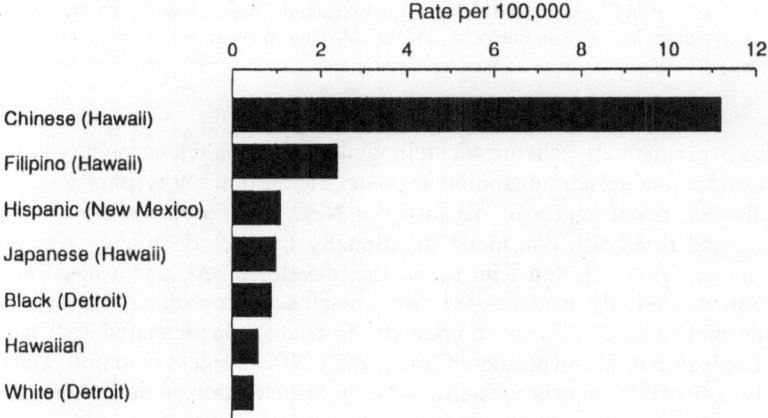

Figure 5. Average annual age-adjusted incidence rates (i.e., to the world population of International Agency for Research on Cancer) per 100,000, cancer of nasopharynx, males by race (United States, 1978–1982).

Table 4. Epidemiologic Features of Nasopharyngeal Carcinoma

Risk Factor	Comments
Age	Among black and white Americans, incidence increases steadily after age 20, until at least 70 years old. Minor peak in incidence in blacks 10–19 years, which is 3.5 times higher than in whites. Rates in whites exceed those in blacks over age 50 years. Incidence in Chinese Americans is about 30 times higher than in whites or blacks, peaking at 50–59 years.
Sex	Rates in men are two to three times higher than in women in all populations studied.
Geography	In the lowest risk countries (e.g., North America, Europe), annual rates are <1/100,000. Intermediate-risk countries (e.g., Malaysia, Thailand, Indonesia, Arab populations in northern Africa, Israeli Jews born in Africa or Asia) rates vary between 2 and 5 per 100,000. Highest risk countries (>5/100,000) include Cantonese Chinese males from southern provinces (30/100,000), as well as Eskimos, Aleuts, and Indians in Alaska (13.5/100,000). Among high-risk southern Chinese, individuals in lower social strata are at higher risk than those in higher social strata.
Epstein-Barr virus (EBV)	There are significantly higher antibody titers to EBV-associated viral capsid, early and nuclear antigens. Antibody levels increase with advancing stages of disease. EBV DNA is integrated in the genome of epithelial cells in tumor tissue. Virtually all Chinese children are infected by age 5; more than a 20-fold variation in incidence of nasopharyngeal carcinoma (NPC) exists within China.
Dietary	Early and repeated exposures to salted, partially decaying fish is traditional among Cantonese raised in southern Chinese culture. Case-control studies suggest significant dose-response with salted fish exposure, and with odds ratios ranging from 2.0 to 4.5 when exposures are multiple, begins soon after weaning, and lasts more than 10 years. Putative carcinogens in Chinese salted fish include volatile nitrosamines and other bacterial mutagens. Similar dietary association was noted in case-control studies in Alaska. Consumption of other salted or fermented indigenous foods containing volatile nitrosamines may be related to increased risk among Arabs of North Africa. Risks may be enhanced with deficient consumption of fresh fruits and vegetables.
Environmental chemicals: fumes, smoke, dust	Occupational and residential (e.g., mobile homes) exposures to formaldehyde have been linked with respiratory tract cancers including NPC, but there have been uncertainties in measuring exposure levels and adjusting for confounders. In contrast to cancer in the oropharynx, larynx, and lung, exposure to tobacco smoke, actively or involuntarily, has not been significantly associated with NPC.
Host factors: HLA genes, genetic markers	Joint occurrence of A2-BW46 antigens associated with twofold increased risk of NPC in southern China. Other HLA antigens implicated in southern Chinese are B17 (AW19-B17), A11, and B13. In contrast to southern Chinese, BW46 is an uncommon antigen haplotype in Europeans and the U.S. white population.

As demonstrated experimentally, chemical carcinogens may reach the nasopharynx by inhalation, ingestion, and parenteral administration. In contrast to the oral cavity, pharynx, and larynx, tobacco and alcohol are not significant risk factors in NPC. It was proposed that among the Cantonese, salted and dried fish consumed traditionally from early infancy was an important etiologic factor (19). Rats fed with salted fish developed malignant nasal and paranasal tumors. Salted, partially decomposed fish contains appreciable quantities of nitrosodimethylamine and other N-nitroso compounds. Consumption of salted fish was unusual as a dietary staple in central and northern China, where NPC was less common. Thus, the complex natural history of NPC may be viewed as a dynamic interaction of viral, chemical, and genetic factors.

Nasal Cavity and Paranasal Sinuses

Cancers of the nasal cavity and paranasal sinuses account for less than 2% of all incidences of respiratory cancers in the United States. Unlike lung cancer, sinonasal cancer incidence does not differ significantly between blacks and whites, and the annual age-adjusted incidence rates, generally less than 1.0 per 100,000, have been relatively stable over the past 25 years. Age-specific incidence rates in females tend to be lower than in males at every age group. Epidemiologic studies have not established a strong causal link between tobacco and alcohol exposures and sinonasal cancer. Carcinoma of the nasal cavity or paranasal sinuses may serve as a "sentinel" for past cumulative exposures to a specific respiratory tract carcinogen associated with the workplace or ambient environment (Table 5) (20–22).

Multiple Primary Cancers

Patients with a previous primary epidermoid carcinoma in the aerodigestive tract are at increased risk of developing metachronous primary cancers in the contiguous mucosal tissue. "Field cancerization" or multicentric SCCs developing in the aerodigestive tract are an important reason for therapeutic failure following treatment of the index primary cancer (23,24). The cumulative incidence of metachronous multiple primary cancers in the aerodigestive tract within 10 years after treatment of the index primary "head and neck" cancer has been reported variously between 5% and 40%, or between 0.5% and 3.5% per year (25).

The bidirectional or mutual nature of elevated risks for multiple primary cancers in subsites in the aerodigestive tract, with the exclusion of the nasopharynx, nasal cavity, and paranasal sinuses, may be attributed to common causal associations with previous consumption levels of tobacco and alcohol (26).

ETIOLOGY

Tobacco

The complexity of tobacco smoke with over 3000 different chemicals has made it difficult to identify the contribution of specific putative carcinogenic agents. The carcinogens in tobacco smoke include the polynuclear aromatic hydrocarbons (benz[a]anthracene, benzo[a]-pyrene), N-nitrosamines (N-nitrosodimethylamine, N'-nitrosonornicotine [NNN]), aromatic amines (2-naphthylamine, 4-aminobiphenyl), aldehydes (formaldehyde, acetaldehyde), other organic (benzene, acrylonitrile) and inorganic (arsenic, chromium) compounds, and polonium 210. The composition of the smoke depends on the ambient conditions of smoking, the blend of tobacco leaf, filtration, additives, paper wrapping, etc. The majority of the components are

Table 5. Carcinomas in Nasal Cavity or Paranasal Sinuses: "Sentinel Cancers" for Exposure to Environmental Agents

---

Nickel refining[a] (metallic nickel, nickel subsulfide, oxide, or carbonyl)
Chromium[a] (hexavalent chromate as in pigment manufacturing)
Ionizing radiation (radium, thorotrast or thorium dioxide)
Mustard-gas[a] manufacturing
Isopropyl alcohol manufacturing[a] (isopropyl oil, diisopropyl sulfate)
Gas manufacture[a] (polycyclic aromatic hydrocarbons)
Furniture and other woodworking (hardwood dusts)
Boot and shoe manufacturing (leather or wood dust constituents)
Textile and clothing manufacturing (wool dust constituents)

---

[a]Respiratory tract carcinogen with associated risks in larynx and lung.

produced in an oxygen-deficient, hydrogen-rich environment, arising from pyrolysis and distillation, in the region immediately behind the burning tip of the cigarette.

The chemical analysis of tobacco smoke is separated into particulate or "tar" and gaseous phases. Filter tips of cellulose acetate remove volatile nitrosamines and phenols selectively. The neutral fraction of the particulate phase contains potentially important tumor initiators, such as the polynuclear aromatic hydrocarbons. The epoxide metabolites of the polynuclear aromatic hydrocarbons bind covalently with DNA and function as genotoxic initiators in a complex multistage process (27).

The curing, fermentation, and aging of smokeless tobacco products (e.g., plug tobacco, loose-leaf tobacco, twist tobacco, and snuff) favor the formation from tobacco alkaloids of various N-nitrosamines. Among the nitrosamines in smokeless tobacco, NNN and 4(methyl-nitrosamino)-1-(3-pyridyl)-1-butanone (NNK) are carcinogenic in variously tested rodents. During chewing or "snuff dipping," additional amounts of carcinogenic tobacco-specific N-nitrosamines are formed endogenously in the oral cavity (28–30).

Epidemiologic studies conducted in many countries have established that the risks of oral cavity, pharyngeal, laryngeal, lung, and esophageal cancers are significantly increased among cigarette smokers. The degree of exposure, as measured by the average number of cigarettes smoked per day, is associated with substantially increasing levels of risk (Table 6). When compared with nonsmokers, a cohort of U.S. male veterans who smoked 40 or more cigarettes per day experienced a relative risk of dying of cancer of the lung that was increased almost 24-fold; larynx, 32-fold; oral cavity, more than 12-fold; and esophagus, more than 9-fold. Exposure to cigar or pipe tobacco was associated with elevated risks of cancer throughout the aerodigestive tract; in particular, cigar tobacco increased the risk of cancer in the larynx and upper digestive organ sites (Table 7) (31).

The degree of exposure and consequential risk will also be affected significantly by the duration of smoking, depth of inhalation, and cigarette tar yield. In the earlier American Cancer Society (ACS) Twenty-five–State Study, males who smoked low-tar and low-nicotine

Table 6. Relative Risk of Mortality from Upper Aerodigestive Tract Cancers Among Men According to Average Number of Cigarettes Smoked[a]

No. Cigarettes Smoked (per day)	Relative Risk[b]			
	Lung	Larynx	Oral Cavity	Esophagus
1–9	5.5	5.3	2.9	3.1
10–20	9.9	9.2	2.9	4.3
21–39	17.4	14.8	6.2	12.4
40+	23.9	32.1	12.4	9.2

[a]Source: Modified from Kahn, U.S. Veterans' Prospective Study (31).
[b]Relative to a risk of 1.0 in men who never smoked regularly.

Table 7. Relative Risk of Mortality from Aerodigestive Tract Cancers Among Men Who Smoke Cigars and Pipes[a]

Smoking Method	Relative Risk[b]			
	Lung	Larynx	Oral Cavity	Esophagus
Cigar only	1.7	10.3	4.1	5.3
Pipe only	2.1	—	3.1	2.0

[a]Source: Modified from Kahn, U.S. Veterans' Prospective Study (31).
[b]Relative to a risk of 1.0 in men who never smoked regularly.

cigarettes experienced a lung cancer mortality rate 20% lower than males who continued to smoke high-tar cigarettes. The excess lung cancer risk for current smokers was directly proportional to the estimated milligrams of tar consumed daily: standardized mortality ratio $= 100 + 1.731 \times$ milligrams of tar per day (32). In the more recent ACS Fifty-State Study, Garfinkel and Stellman concluded that doubling the cigarette tar yield would result in a 40% increase in the relative risk of dying of lung cancer, independently of the amount smoked or depth of inhalation (33).

Further evidence of the etiologic role of tobacco is based on the reduction of risk following cessation of smoking. For example, after 10 years of smoking cessation, the risk of lung cancer is reduced to about 50% of the risk experienced by those of similar age and sex who continue to smoke (Table 8) (34,35). The rate of decline in the excessive risk of dying of lung cancer is influenced by the history of duration of smoking. For example, after 15 years of cigarette smoking, the excess annual incidence rate of lung cancer, or that which is above the background rate in nonsmokers, would be about 1 per 10,000; among those who have smoked 45 years, the excess annual incidence would be about 50 per 10,000. The cumulative lifetime incidence rate of lung cancer in men who have smoked regularly 10–20 cigarettes per day would be about 10%; in those who have smoked regularly 21–39 cigarettes per day, the cumulative incidence rate of lung cancer would be about 20% (36,37). Smoking cessation for at least 5 years will result in risk reduction for incurring cancers throughout the aerodigestive tract (Tables 8 and 9). However, as demonstrated in the studies of U.S. veterans (31) and British physicians (38), even among former smokers who had stopped for 15 years, there was a residually elevated risk of lung cancer that was 2–4 times higher than that in nonsmokers. For those aerodigestive organ sites affected by tobacco and alcohol exposures, former smokers experienced at least a 50% reduction in risk, even after adjusting for prior alcohol consumption (39).

Among women in North Carolina who dipped snuff, there was a fourfold increase in the risk of oral cancer. In particular, among the long-term users, the relative risk reached nearly 50 for SCCs arising in the gingivobuccal sulcus, where there was prolonged contact with the snuff tobacco powder. The authors estimated that 87% of the cancers of the oral and gingival mucosa in the southeastern United States were due to snuff use (40).

In countries such as India, China, Pakistan, Thailand, Sri Lanka, Afghanistan, and Central Republic of the Soviet Union, where the use of snuff and chewing tobacco are quite common, oral and pharyngeal cancer mortality rates are among the highest in the world. For example, use of smokeless tobacco in India and Southeast Asia involves preparing a betel quid consisting of the leaf of the betel vine (Piper betle), sliced or shaved areca nut from the betel palm (Areca catechu), and powdered slaked lime. One or more additives (e.g., gambier, catechu, cardamom, cloves, aniseed), with or without tobacco, complete the preparation of the

Table 8. Cigarette Smoking Cessation Benefits in Case-Control Studies of Male Patients with Squamous Cell Carcinomas[a]

Smoking Status	Relative Risk			
	Lung	Larynx	Oral Cavity	Esophagus
Never smoked	1.0	1.0	1.0	1.0
Current smoker	32.3	14.3	8.9	3.6
Former smoker:				
1–3 yrs since stopping	53.8	17.9	9.0	4.8
4–6 yrs since stopping	24.9	8.5	3.5	1.5
7–10 yrs since stopping	17.2	4.0	3.2	1.4
11–15 yrs since stopping	13.7	3.4	3.4	1.3
≥16 yrs since stopping	5.0	2.5	1.6	1.0

[a]Source: Modified from Wynder and Stellman (34).

Table 9. American Cancer Society Prospective Study II: Age-standardized Mortality Ratios[a] for Aerodigestive Tract Cancer by Baseline Cigarette Smoking Status[b]

Cancer Site	Sex[c]	Current Smoker	Former Smoker
Oral cavity	M	27.5	8.8
	F	5.6	2.9
Larynx	M	10.5	5.2
	F	17.8	11.9
Lung	M	22.4	9.4
	F	11.9	5.0
Esophagus	M	7.6	5.8
	F	10.3	3.2

[a]Ratio of age-adjusted death rates, where age adjustment was based upon the age distribution of person-years among male and female nonsmokers. The referent group never smoked, with risk of 1.0.
[b]Source: Modified from Garfinkel and Stellman (33).
[c]Patients were 35 years of age and older.

betel quid, which is then chewed. Protracted use is associated with the pathologic sequelae of erythroleukoplakia, epithelial dysplasia, and, ultimately, epidermoid carcinoma of the gingivo-buccal or lingual mucosa, hypopharynx, supraglottis, or esophagus (41,42).

Alcohol

Ethanol appears to enhance the carcinogenic effects of N-nitrosodimethylamine in tissues of the nasal cavity, upper digestive tract, and lung, when administered orally to mice. Ethanol has a selective effect on the toxicity of N-nitrosodimethylamine by inducing the cytochrome P-450 system, which functions as a nitrosodimethylamine demethylase. Induction by ethanol of the cytochrome P-450–dependent microsomal oxidizing system, derived from the liver, lung, and upper digestive tract, may serve to enhance susceptibility to and activation of chemical procarcinogens. Chemicals such as ethanol may accelerate the microsomal degradation of vitamin A, resulting in hepatic depletion of retinol (43,44).

Various oxidative pathways of ethanol metabolism result in the production of acetaldehyde. Acetaldehyde is a reactive compound that forms adducts with various proteins, interferes with DNA repair, induces sister chromatid exchanges, and promotes depletion of glutathione, toxicity mediated by free radicals and lipid peroxidation (45). Minute amounts of acetaldehyde inactivate O^6-methylguanine transferase, the enzyme responsible for repairing adducts resulting from alkylation at the O^6 position of guanine.

When ethanol is applied topically to buccal, nasal, or rectal mucosa, or skin, or when given orally as part of the diet, it has a cocarcinogenic effect when administered in conjunction with a genotoxic agent such as 7,12-dimethylbenz[a]anthracene, diethylnitrosamine, nitrosopyrrolidine, or dimethylhydrazine. The local cytotoxic and solvent actions of ethanol may result in enhanced mucosal cell damage and permeability, followed by reparative basal epithelial cell proliferation. The association of ethanol ingestion with the induction of cancers at sites that are not in direct contact with the agent would require the participation of systemic ethanol-dependent mechanisms.

Congeners or contaminants identified in ethanol of potential significance in human carcinogenesis include the nitrosamines (e.g., N-nitrosodimethylamine); polycyclic, aromatic hydrocarbons (e.g., phenanthrene, benz[a]anthracene, benzo[a]pyrene); aromatic and aliphatic fusel oils; and other mutagenic compounds. Locally prepared alcoholic beverages, indigenous to a particular culture or geographic region, are more likely than commercially prepared beverages to contain measurable quantities at approximate levels of 1–3 parts per billion of toxic contaminants. A proposed schematic summary of putative mechanisms for the carcinogenic actions of ethanol is presented in Figure 6.

Epidemiologic studies demonstrate that the ingestion of alcohol increases independently the risks of incurring epidermoid carcinomas of the upper aerodigestive tract (46,47). Because alcohol and tobacco are generally consumed jointly, the relative risks are presented for the combined exposures (Tables 10–12) (44,48,49). Of biologic and public health significance is the demonstration of potentiation of risk by the multiplicative interaction of increasing levels of exposure to both agents. For oral and pharyngeal cancer, joint exposure to tobacco and alcohol results in odds ratios that are 2–2.5 times those expected if the effects of alcohol and tobacco were only additive (Table 10) (48). For laryngeal cancer, Flanders and Rothman concluded that the interaction of alcohol and tobacco increases the risk about 50% more than the increase predicted if the effects were only additive (50). The subsites within the upper aerodigestive tract exhibiting interaction with previous ethanol exposure are the floor of mouth, hypopharynx, supraglottis, and esophagus (51–53). Combined exposures to alcohol and tobacco in the United States account for 75–85% of the incident cancers of the oral cavity, pharynx, larynx and esophagus.

Antioxidant Micronutrients

A number of nutritional factors are thought to be important as modifiers of aerodigestive tract carcinogenesis. In the United States, nutritional deficiencies are commonly associated with, or exacerbated by, excessive alcohol ingestion. The potential interactions of deficiencies in essential micronutrients and exogenous genotoxic agents may give rise to altered mucosal integrity, enzyme and metabolic dysfunction, and morphologic abnormalities in specific target organs (54).

Vitamin A and its provitamin, β-carotene, are needed for normal growth and differentiation of epithelial tissues, presumably mediated by regulating gene expression and transcription. Deficiency of vitamin A leads to a loss of mucociliary epithelium in the respiratory tract and its replacement by metaplastic squamous epithelium. The antioxidant micronutrients, such as the carotenoids and vitamin C, serve to trap free radicals and reactive oxygen molecules, which are generated endogenously. Free radicals are highly reactive and attack the

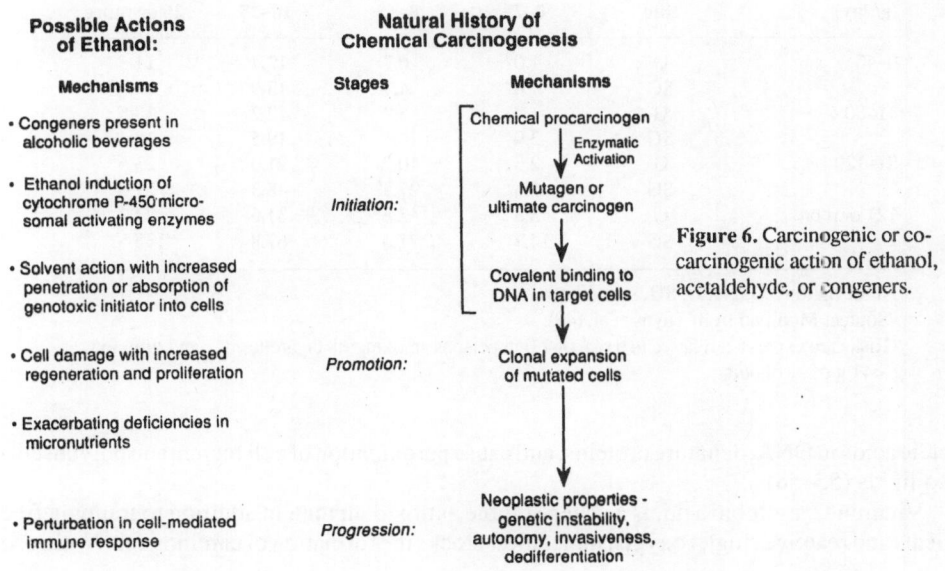

Figure 6. Carcinogenic or co-carcinogenic action of ethanol, acetaldehyde, or congeners.

13

Table 10. Relative Risk of Oral Cavity Cancer Associated with Varying Levels of Exposure to Alcohol and Smoking Tobacco[a]

Alcohol (ozs/day)	Cigarette Equivalents/Day			
	0	1–19	20–39	40 or more
0	1.0[b]	1.5	1.4	2.4
<0.4	1.4	1.7	3.2	3.3
0.4–1.5	1.6	4.4	4.5	8.2
>1.5	2.3	4.1	9.6	15.5

[a]Source: Modified from Rothman and Keller (48).
[b]Risks are expressed relative to risk of 1.0 for persons who neither smoked nor drank.

Table 11. Relative Risk of Esophageal Cancer Associated with Varying Levels of Exposure to Alcohol and Smoking Tobacco[a]

Alcohol (g/day)	Grams of Tobacco Smoked/Day			
	0–9	10–19	20–29	30 or more
0–40	1.0[b]	3.4	3.2	7.8
41–80	7.3	8.4	8.8	35.0
81–120	11.8	13.6	12.6	83.0
121 or more	49.6	65.9	137.6	155.6

[a]Source: Modified from Tuyns et al. (44).
[b]Risks are expressed relative to a risk of 1.0 in persons smoking <10 g of tobacco/day and drinking <41 g of alcohol/day.

Table 12. Relative Risk of Laryngeal Cancer, Comparing Glottis and Supraglottis, Associated with Varying Levels of Exposure to Alcohol and Smoking Tobacco[a]

Alcohol (g/day)	Anatomic Site	Cigarettes Smoked/Day			
		0–7	8–15	16–25	26 or more
0–40	G	1.0[b]	6.7	12.7	11.5
	SG	1.0	4.7	13.9	14.9
41–80	G	1.7	5.9	12.2	18.5
	SG	3.0	14.6	19.5	18.4
81–120	G	2.3	10.7	21.0	23.6
	SG	5.5	27.5	48.3	37.6
121 or more	G	3.8	12.2	31.6	43.2
	SG	14.7	71.6	67.8	135.5

Abbreviations: G, glottis; SG, supraglottis.
[a]Source: Modified from Tuyns et al. (49).
[b]Risks are expressed relative to a risk of 1.0 in persons smoking <8 cigarettes/day and drinking <41 g of alcohol/day.

nucleic acids in DNA, denature proteins, and cause peroxidation of cell membrane polyunsaturated lipids (55–58).

Vitamin C, ascorbic acid, is a water-soluble antioxidant that, in addition to trapping free radicals and reactive singlet oxygen molecules, blocks the formation of carcinogenic N-nitroso compounds. The substrate or precursors for these compounds may be derived from tobacco, foods, and food additives (e.g., nitrite-cured meats and salted, pickled, or smoked fish or meat); alcoholic beverages; or pharmaceuticals. The primary dietary sources of vitamin C are fruits and vegetables, especially citrus fruits, green leafy vegetables, tomatoes, and potatoes (59–61).

Vitamin A in foods may occur as preformed vitamin A, namely, retinol and retinol esters derived from animal foods, or as provitamin A carotenoids derived from plant foods, which can be converted to vitamin A. There are many other naturally occurring carotenoids in fruits and vegetables, however, that are not precursors of vitamin A, but are effective antioxidants and efficient scavengers of reactive oxygen molecules. Foods such as green and orange-yellow vegetables are a rich source of carotenoids, containing 600 mcg or more of carotene per 100 g of edible parts, in addition to vitamin C, calcium, iron, and dietary fiber.

The most compelling information on the relative protective effects of consumption of fresh vegetables in individuals who smoke has been in patients with lung cancer. In a cohort study conducted by Hirayama in Japan, daily consumption of fresh green-yellow vegetables lowered the relative risk of lung cancer mortality in men who smoked 25 or more cigarettes per day by at least 40% when compared with individuals with comparable cigarette smoking exposure who rarely or never consumed fresh vegetables (62). Among ex-smokers, the rate of reduction in the risk of dying of lung cancer after adjusting for previous smoking history was enhanced among men who were daily consumers of green-yellow vegetables, when compared with those who rarely or never consumed fresh vegetables. Most, but not all, case-control and cohort studies conducted in men and women described increases in relative risk ranging from 1.3 to 7.2, after adjusting for cigarette smoking, for individuals in the lowest tertile or quartile of consumption of green-yellow vegetables or of vitamin A or carotene, as determined from food composition tables (63–65). Analyses of histologic type showed protective effects in relation to squamous and small cell carcinomas of the lung when frequency of consumption of vegetables or carotenoids was measured; the inverse relationship with adenocarcinoma was also established, although not as consistently. Serum carotenoids, or specifically serum β-carotene levels, were generally found to vary inversely with the risk of lung cancer. The cigarette smoking–adjusted odds ratios for developing lung cancer ranged from 2.0 to 2.3 for those in the lowest versus the highest levels of serum β-carotene (66,67).

Infrequent consumption of fresh fruits and vegetables was noted in populations throughout the world at increased risk of esophageal cancer. In a study of black males with esophageal cancer in the United States, food frequency consumption at the lowest tertile for vegetables and fruits, and of nutrient sources of vitamin C, was associated with twofold increases in relative risk after adjusting for tobacco and ethanol consumption (Table 13) (68). Of five case-control studies that estimated vegetable sources for total dietary carotenoids or vitamin A, three detected an inverse association with esophageal cancer (69–71). Case-control studies have provided support for a protective effect of vitamin C, of dietary carotenoids, of fresh citrus fruits, or of green leafy vegetables, on the relative risk of oral and pharyngeal cancers. Smoking- and alcohol-adjusted odds ratios for low consumption of dietary vitamin C or of fresh fruits, as compared with high consumption levels, have ranged from 1.7 to 2.5 in studies of patients with oral and pharyngeal cancers (72).

Animal and epidemiologic studies have provided the rationale for developing and testing chemopreventive agents, generally comprised of natural or synthetic analogues of micronutrients, which may inhibit or reverse the carcinogenic process. The various mechanisms of action expressed by chemopreventive agents include 1) inducing metabolic detoxification of proximate or ultimate carcinogens; 2) scavenging reactive singlet oxygen molecules and free radicals; and 3) inducing epithelial cell differentiation and reversing preneoplastic morphologic lesions (73–75). In a controlled clinical trial conducted in patients who were disease-free after undergoing primary treatment for SCCs of the oral cavity, pharynx, or larynx, the random assignment of patients to receive daily oral isotretinoin (13-*cis*–retinoic acid) resulted, after

Table 13. Adjusted Relative Risks[a] of Esophageal Cancer in U.S. Black Males by Food Group and Micronutrient Intake[b]

Food Group	Level of Consumption (Tertiles)			
	Highest	Middle	Lowest	P (trend)
Complex carbohydrates	1.0	1.1	1.2	0.24
Meat and fish	1.0	1.3	1.2	0.39
Vegetables	1.0	1.5	1.6	0.07
Fruits	1.0	2.4	2.0	0.05
Vegetables and fruits	1.0	1.7	2.0	0.02
Vitamin A	1.0	1.5	1.5	0.10
Carotenoids	1.0	1.3	1.3	0.17
Vitamin C	1.0	1.2	1.8	0.03
Thiamine	1.0	1.2	1.2	0.34

[a]Adjusted for tobacco and ethanol consumption.
[b]Source: Modified from Ziegler et al. (68).

a median follow-up of 32 months, in the cumulative incidence of second primary cancers of 24% in the placebo group, as compared with 4% in the treatment group ($P = 0.005$) (76). The administration of β-carotene alone or in combination with vitamin A in individuals who chew the betel nut quid with tobacco can decrease the incidence of new lesions of leukoplakia in the oral mucosa or the incidence of micronucleated cells in exfoliated oral mucosal cells (77–79). The micronucleated cells are an intermediate endpoint marker of genotoxic damage produced by carcinogens (80).

Host Factors

Genetically determined clinical disorders, or even more subtle metabolic dysfunctional phenotypes, can be demonstrated to alter susceptibility to environmental mutagens. The carcinogenic process may be viewed as a complex and dynamic interaction of environment and heredity. Indeed, "ecogenetics," or the study of genetic variability in response to specific environmental agents, is analogous to the concern in pharmacogenetics of host variability with respect to therapeutic response, toxicity, and detoxification of any pharmaceutical agent (81). The ultimate outcome of exposure to mutagens and clastogens will depend on competitive gene-enzyme interactions or on the integrity of endogenous mechanisms for repairing lesions in DNA and affecting the cascade of immunologic responses.

Oral and pharyngeal cancer patients have been reported to have increased sensitivity to chromosome damage from clastogens, independent of their tobacco and alcohol habits (82). In some rare inherited genodermatoses, which are associated with high epithelial cell turnover and abnormal DNA repair, there is increased susceptibility for developing skin, oropharyngeal, and esophageal cancers. These clinical disorders include X-linked dyskeratosis congenita, ectodermal dysplasia, epidermolysis bullosa, xeroderma pigmentosum, Bloom syndrome, and tylosis (83,84).

A genetically controlled ability to metabolize the antihypertensive agent debrisoquine has been linked to the risk of contracting lung cancer. For example, individuals who metabolize debrisoquine extensively, as determined by the rate of urinary excretion of 4-hydroxydebrisoquine, are at significantly greater risk of contracting lung cancer than those who metabolize the agent poorly or intermediately. The gene locus responsible for metabolizing debrisoquine produces a specific human isozyme, P-450dbl, which may be directly involved in the carcinogenic process or serve as a genetic linkage marker for susceptibility to tobacco-induced lung cancers (85,86).

REFERENCES

1. American Cancer Society. Cancer Facts and Figures, 1990.
2. Gloeckler-Ries LA, Hankey BF, Edwards BK. Cancer Statistics Review 1973–1987. U.S. Department of Health and Human Services, National Cancer Institute, NIH Publication No. 90–2789.
3. Moore C, Catlin D. Anatomic origins and locations of oral cancer. Am J Surg 114:510–513, 1967.
4. Muir C, Waterhouse J, Mack T, Powell J, Whelan S. Cancer Incidence in Five Continents (Vol. V). Lyon, International Agency for Research on Cancer, Scientific Publication No. 88, 1987.
5. Schottenfeld D. Epidemiology of cancer of the esophagus. Semin Oncol 11:92–100, 1984.
6. Blot WJ, Devesa SS, Kneller RW, Fraumeni JF Jr. Rising incidence of adenocarcinoma of the esophagus and gastric cardia. JAMA 265:1287–1289, 1991.
7. Sartori S, Nielsen I, Indelli M, Trevisani L, Pazzi P, Grandi E. Barrett's esophagus after chemotherapy with cyclophosphamide, methotrexate, and 5-fluorouracil (CMF): An iatrogenic injury. Ann Intern Med 114:210–211, 1991.
8. Yang PC, Thomas DB, Daling JR, David S. Differences in the sex ratio of laryngeal cancer incidence rates by anatomic subsite. J Clin Epidemiol 42:755–758, 1989.
9. Devesa SS, Blot WJ, Fraumeni JF Jr. Cohort trends in mortality from oral, esophageal and laryngeal cancers in the United States. Epidemiology 1:116–121, 1990.
10. McMichael AJ. Increases in laryngeal cancer in Britain and Australia in relation to alcohol and tobacco consumption trends. Lancet 1:1244–1247, 1978.
11. Novotny TE, Warner KE, Kendrick JS, Remington PL. Smoking by blacks and whites: Socioeconomic and demographic differences. Am J Public Health 78:1187–1189, 1988.
12. Walker WJ, Brin BN. United States lung cancer mortality and declining cigarette tobacco consumption. J Clin Epidemiol 41:179–185, 1988.
13. Garfinkel L, Stellman SD. Smoking and lung cancer in women: Findings in a prospective study. Cancer Res 48:6951–6955, 1988.
14. Centers for Disease Control. Cigarette smoking—Behavioral risk factor surveillance system. MMWR 38:845–848, 1989.
15. Escobedo LG, Anda RF, Smith PF, Remington PL, Mast EE. Sociodemographic characteristics of cigarette smoking initiation in the United States. Implications for smoking prevention policy. JAMA 264:1550–1555, 1990.
16. Yu MC, Henderson BF. Nasopharynx. In Schottenfeld D, Fraumeni JF Jr (eds): Cancer Epidemiology and Prevention. 2d ed. New York: Oxford University Press, in press.
17. Pagano JS. Epstein-Barr virus transcription in nasopharyngeal carcinoma. J Virol 48:580–589, 1983.
18. Henle W, Henle G. Epstein-Barr virus and human malignancies. Advances in Viral Oncology 5:201–238, 1985.
19. Ning J-P, Yu MC, Wang Q-S, Henderson BE. Consumption of salted fish and other risk factors for nasopharyngeal carcinoma (NPC) in Tianjin, a low-risk region for NPC in the People's Republic of China. J Natl Cancer Inst 82:291–296, 1990.
20. Frank AL. Occupational cancers of the respiratory system. Seminars in Occupational Medicine 2:257–266, 1987.
21. Vaughan TL, Davis S. Wood dust exposure and squamous cell cancers of the upper respiratory tract. Am J Epidemiol 133:560–564, 1991.
22. Roush GC. Nasal cavity and paranasal sinuses. In Schottenfeld D, Fraumeni JF Jr (eds): Cancer Epidemiology and Prevention. 2d ed. New York: Oxford University Press, in press.
23. Slaughter DP, Southwick HW, Smejkal W. "Field cancerization" in oral stratified squamous epithelium: Clinical implications of multicentric origin. Cancer 6:963–968, 1953.
24. Strong MS, Incze J, Vaughan CW. Field cancerization in the aerodigestive tract: Its etiology, manifestation and significance. J Otolaryngol 13:1–6, 1984.
25. Winn DM, Blot WJ. Second cancers following cancers of the buccal cavity and pharynx in Connecticut, 1935–1982. In National Cancer Institute Monograph no. 68. Washington, D.C.: Government Printing Office, 1985, pp. 25–48 (NIH publication no. 85-2714).
26. Schottenfeld D, Gantt RC, Wynder EL. The role of alcohol and tobacco in multiple primary cancers of the upper digestive system, larynx and lung: A prospective study. Prev Med 3:277–293, 1974.
27. Jeffrey PK. Tobacco smoke-induced lung disease. In Cohen RD, Lewis B, Alberti KGMM, Denman AM (eds): The Metabolic and Molecular Basis of Acquired Disease. London: Bailliere, Tindall, 1990, pp. 466–495.
28. Hoffmann D, Hecht SS. Nicotine-derived N-nitrosamines and tobacco-related cancer: Current status and future directions. Cancer Res 45:935–944, 1985.
29. Hoffmann D, Adams JD, Lisk D, Fisenne I, Brunnemann KD. Toxic and carcinogenic agents in dry and moist snuff. J Natl Cancer Inst 79:1281–1286, 1987.
30. Hecht SS, Hoffmann D. The relevance of tobacco-specific nitrosamines to human cancer. Cancer Surv 8:273–294, 1989.

31. Kahn HA. The Dorn study on smoking and mortality among U.S. veterans: Report on 8-1/2 years of observation. In Haenszel W (ed): Epidemiological Approaches to the Study of Cancer and Other Chronic Diseases. National Cancer Institute Monograph no. 19. Bethesda, MD, 1966, pp. 1–125.

32. Stellman SD, Garfinkel L. Lung cancer risk is proportional to cigarette tar yield: Evidence from a prospective study. Prev Med 18:518–525, 1989.

33. Stellman SD, Garfinkel L. Smoking habits and tar levels in a new American Cancer Society prospective study of 1.2 million men and women. J Natl Cancer Inst 76:1057–1063, 1986.

34. Wynder EL, Stellman SD. Comparative epidemiology of tobacco-related cancers. Cancer Res 37:4608–4622, 1977.

35. U.S. Department of Health and Human Services. The Health Benefits of Smoking Cessation: A Report of the Surgeon General, Centers for Disease Control, Center for Chronic Disease Prevention and Health Promotion, Office on Smoking and Health, DHHS Publication No. (CDC) 90-8416, 1990.

36. Peto R. Influence of dose and duration of smoking on lung cancer rates. In Zaridze DG, Peto R (eds): Tobacco: A Major International Health Hazard. Lyon: International Agency for Research on Cancer, 1986, pp. 23–33.

37. Doll R, Peto R. Cigarette smoking and bronchial carcinoma: Dose and time relationships among regular smokers and life-long nonsmokers. J Epidemiol Community Health 32:303–313, 1978.

38. Doll R, Peto R. Mortality in relation to smoking: 20 Years' observations on male British doctors. Br Med J 2:1525–1536, 1976.

39. Freedman DA, Navidi WC. Ex-smokers and multistage model for lung cancer. Epidemiology 1:21–29, 1990.

40. Winn DM, Blot WJ, Shy CM, Pickle LW, Toledo A, Fraumeni JF Jr. Snuff dipping and oral cancer among women in the southern United States. N Engl J Med 304:745–749, 1981.

41. International Agency for Research on Cancer. IARC Monographs on the Evaluation of the Carcinogenic Risk of Chemicals to Humans: Tobacco Habits Other Than Smoking; Betel Quid and Areca Nut Chewing; and Some Related Nitrosamines, vol. 37. Lyon: World Health Organization, 1985.

42. Gupta PC, Pindborg JJ, Mehta FS. Comparison of carcinogenicity of betel quid with and without tobacco: An epidemiological review. Ecology and Disease 1:213–219, 1982.

43. Lieber CS. Biochemical and molecular basis of alcohol-induced injury to liver and other tissues. N Engl J Med 319:1639–1650, 1988.

44. International Agency for Research on Cancer. Alcohol Drinking. IARC Monographs on the Evaluation of Carcinogenic Risks to Humans, vol. 44. Lyon: World Health Organization, 1988.

45. Obe G, Ristow H. Acetaldehyde but not alcohol induces sister chromatid exchanges in Chinese hamster cells in vitro. Mutat Res 56:211–213, 1977.

46. Kissin B. Epidemiologic investigation of possible biological interactions of alcohol and cancer of the head and neck. Ann N Y Acad Sci 252:374–384, 1975.

47. Schottenfeld D. Alcohol as a co-factor in the etiology of cancer. Cancer 43:1962–1966, 1979.

48. Rothman K, Keller AZ. The effect of joint exposure to alcohol and tobacco on risk of cancer of the mouth and pharynx. Journal of Chronic Disease 25:711–716, 1972.

49. Tuyns AJ, Esteve J, Raymond L, Berrino F, Benhamou E, Blanchet F, Boffetta P, Crosignani P, del Moral A, Lehmann W, Merletti F, Pequignot G, Riboli E, Sancho-Garnier H, Terracini B, Zubiri A, Zubiri Z. Cancer of the larynx/hypopharynx, tobacco and alcohol. Int J Cancer 41:483–491, 1988.

50. Flanders WD, Rothman KJ. Interaction of alcohol and tobacco in laryngeal cancer. Am J Epidemiol 115:371–379, 1982.

51. Notani PN. Role of alcohol in cancers of the upper alimentary tract: Use of models in risk assessment. J Epidemiol Community Health 42:187–192, 1988.

52. Blot WJ, McLaughlin JK, Winn DM, Austin DF, Greenberg RS, Preston-Martin S, Bernstein L, Schoenberg JB, Stemhagen A, Fraumeni JF Jr. Smoking and drinking in relation to oral pharyngeal cancer. Cancer Res 48:3282–3287, 1988.

53. LaVecchia C, Negri E. The role of alcohol in esophageal cancer in non-smokers, and the role of tobacco in non-drinkers. Int J Cancer 43:784–785, 1989.

54. Micozzi MS. Foods, micronutrients, and reduction of human cancer. In Moon TE, Micozzi MS (eds): Nutrition and Cancer Prevention: Investigating the Role of Micronutrients. New York: Marcel Dekker, 1989, pp. 213–241.

55. Peto R, Doll R, Buckley JD, Sporn MB. Can dietary beta-carotene materially reduce cancer rates? Nature 290:201–208, 1981.

56. Krinsky NI, Deneke SM. Interaction of oxygen and oxy-radicals with carotenoids. J Natl Cancer Inst 69:205–209, 1982.

57. Lippman SM, Meyskens FL Jr. Retinoids for the prevention of cancer. In Moon TE, Micozzi MS (eds): Nutrition and Cancer Prevention: Investigating the Role of Micronutrients. New York: Marcel Dekker, 1989, pp. 243–271.

58. Garewal HS. Potential role of beta-carotene in prevention of oral cancer. Am J Clin Nutr 53:294S–297S, 1991.

59. Mirvish SS. Blocking the formation of N-nitroso compounds with ascorbic acid in vitro and in vivo. Ann N Y Acad Sci 258:175–180, 1975.

60. Block G, Menkes M. Ascorbic acid in cancer prevention. In Moon TE, Micozzi MS (eds): Nutrition and Cancer Prevention: Investigating the Role of Micronutrients. New York: Marcel Dekker, 1989, pp. 341–388.
61. Block G. Vitamin C and cancer prevention: The epidemiologic evidence. Am J Clin Nutr 53:270S–282S, 1991.
62. Hirayama T. Life-Style and Mortality. Basel: Karger, 1990, pp. 73–95.
63. Bjelke E. Dietary vitamin A and human lung cancer. Int J Cancer 15:561–565, 1975.
64. Kvale G, Bjelke E, Gart JJ. Dietary habits and lung cancer risk. Int J Cancer 31:397–405, 1983.
65. Pisani P, Berrino F, Macaluso M, Pastorino U, Crosignani P, Baldasseroni A. Carrots, green vegetables and lung cancer: A case-control study. Int J Epidemiol 15:463–468, 1986.
66. Wald NJ, Boreham J, Bailey A. Serum retinol and subsequent risk of cancer. Br J Cancer 54:957–961, 1986.
67. Pastorino U, Pisani P, Berrino F, Andreoli C, Barbieri A, Costa A, Mazzoleni C, Gramegna G, Marubini E. Vitamin A and female lung cancer: A case-control study on plasma and diet. Nutr Cancer 10:171–179, 1987.
68. Ziegler RG, Morris LE, Blot WJ, Pottern LM, Hoover R, Fraumeni JF Jr. Esophageal cancer among black men in Washington, D.C. II. Role of nutrition. J Natl Cancer Inst 67:1199–1206, 1981.
69. Tuyns AJ, Riboli E, Doornbos G, Pequignot G. Diet and esophageal cancer in Calvados (France). Nutr Cancer 9:81–92, 1987.
70. Decarli A, Liati P, Negri E, Franceschi S, LaVecchia C. Vitamin A and other dietary factors in the etiology of esophageal cancer. Nutr Cancer 10:29–37, 1987.
71. Graham S, Marshall J, Haughey B, Brasure J, Freudenheim J, Zielezny M, Wilkinson G, Nolan J. Nutritional epidemiology of cancer of the esophagus. Am J Epidemiol 131:454–467, 1990.
72. McLaughlin JK, Gridley G, Block G, Winn DM, Preston-Martin S, Schoenberg JB, Greenberg RS, Stemhagen A, Austin DF, Ershow AG, Blot WJ, Fraumeni JF Jr. Dietary factors in oral and pharyngeal cancer. J Natl Cancer Inst 80:1237–1243, 1988.
73. Wattenberg LW. Chemoprevention of cancer. Cancer Res 45:1–8, 1985.
74. Boone CW, Kelloff GJ, Malone WE. Identification of candidate cancer chemopreventive agents and their evaluation in animal models and human clinical trials: A review. Cancer Res 50:2–9, 1990.
75. Meyskens FL. Coming of age—The chemoprevention of cancer. N Engl J Med 323:825–827 1990.
76. Hong WK, Lippman SM, Itri LM, Karp DD, Lee JS, Byers RM, Schantz SP, Kramer AM, Lotan R, Peters LJ, Dimery IW, Brown BW, Goepfert H. Prevention of second primary tumors with isotretinoin in squamous-cell carcinoma of the head and neck. N Engl J Med 323:795–801, 1990.
77. Shirname LP, Menon MM, Bhide SV. Mutagenicity of betel quid and its ingredients using mammalian test systems. Carcinogenesis 5:501–503, 1984.
78. Stich HF, Rosin MP, Hornby AP, Mathew B, Sankaranarayanan R, Nair MK. Remission of oral leukoplakias and micronuclei in tobacco/betel quid chewers treated with beta-carotene and with beta-carotene plus vitamin A. Int J Cancer 42:195–199, 1988.
79. Stich HF, Mathew B, Sankaranarayanan R, Nair MK. Remission of precancerous lesions in the oral cavity of tobacco chewers and maintenance of the protective effect of beta-carotene or vitamin A. Am J Clin Nutr 53:298S–304S, 1991.
80. Lippman SM, Lee JS, Lotan R, Hittelman W, Wargovich MJ, Hong WK. Biomarkers as intermediate endpoints in chemoprevention trials. J Natl Cancer Inst 82:555–560, 1990.
81. Mulvihill JJ. Host factors in human lung tumors: An example of ecogenetics in oncology. J Natl Cancer Inst 57:3–7, 1976.
82. Spitz MR, Fueger JJ, Beddingfield NA, Annegers JF, Hsu TC, Newell GR, Schantz SP. Chromosome sensitivity to bleomycin-induced mutagenesis, an independent risk factor for upper aerodigestive tract cancers. Cancer Res 49:4626–4628, 1989.
83. Tyldesley WR. Oral leukoplakia associated with tylosis and esophageal carcinoma. J Oral Pathol 3:62–70, 1974.
84. O'Mahony MY, Ellis JP, Hellier M, Mann R, Huddy P. Familial tylosis and carcinoma of the oesophagus. J R Soc Med 77:514–517, 1984.
85. Iannuzzi MC, Miller YE. Genetic predisposition to lung cancer. Seminars in Respiratory Medicine 7.327–332, 1986.
86. Caporaso NE, Tucker MA, Hoover RN, Hayes RB, Pickle LW, Issaq HJ, Muschik GM, Green-Gallo L, Buivys D, Aisner S, Resau JH, Trump BF, Tollerud D, Ainsley W, Harris CC. Lung cancer and the debrisoquine metabolic phenotype. J Natl Cancer Inst 82:1264–1272, 1990.

Epidemiology of Vitamin A and Aerodigestive Cancer

Curtis J. Mettlin

Roswell Park Memorial Institute
Buffalo, New York

During the last decade, there has been a steady progression of research on the dietary epidemiology of aerodigestive cancers, particularly as it relates to vitamin A and its precursor β-carotene. The research, which has involved multiple investigators employing a wide range of research strategies and has concerned several different tumor types and populations at risk, has made epidemiologic findings with implications for further research and public health intervention. The bulk of this research has centered on lung, esophageal, oral, and laryngeal cancers, and this research will be discussed below.

LUNG CANCER

Cigarette smoking is perhaps the most significant human carcinogen, and its association with the twentieth-century epidemic of lung cancer in the United States is well established. However, because individual responses to common levels of cigarette-smoke exposure are variable, several other factors have been investigated as agents that enhance or impede the carcinogenic potential of tobacco smoke. By the mid-1970s, animal experimentation had shown that manipulation of vitamin A exposure affected the susceptibility of rodents to respiratory tract carcinogens (1). Vitamin A in the human diet is obtained principally by consumption of its precursor β-carotene in fruits and vegetables. Two early prospective studies by Hirayama in Japan (2) and Bjelke (3) in Norway, respectively, showed that persons who reported infrequent consumption of foods that are major sources of dietary vitamin A subsequently experienced a greater risk of lung cancer than persons with greater vitamin A intake.

Prospective epidemiologic studies have the advantage of documenting exposure prior to the onset of disease, but have the disadvantage of requiring that large populations be observed over several years to accrue sufficient occurrences of cancer for analysis. For common cancers, retrospective studies have the advantage of being able to study large numbers of persons with disease in relatively short study periods. Development of strategies to study vitamin A and lung cancer retrospectively in human populations provided a significant stimulus to research on the topic. MacLennan et al. (4) and Mettlin and colleagues (5) showed that lung cancer patients were approximately half as likely as other persons with similar life-styles to report low intake of foods that typically are sources of vitamin A. In the study by Mettlin et al., the evidence suggested that there was a gradient of risk correlated with the level of β-carotene intake, and

The Biology and Prevention of Aerodigestive Tract Cancers
Edited by G.R.Newell and W.K. Hong, Plenum Press, New York, 1992

21

this was interpreted as consistent with the hypothesis of a dose-response relationship between vitamin A and lung cancer. This particular study was repeated at Roswell Park Memorial Institute (Buffalo, NY) recently; the dose-response nature of this association is depicted in Figure 1 (6). Men in the highest quintile of β-carotene intake had half the risk of lung cancer as men with the lowest levels of self-reported consumption, a significant risk reduction.

This adaptation of the retrospective research strategy made it possible for many studies of the β-carotene/lung cancer hypothesis to be replicated by several investigators in different settings relatively quickly. Since the earliest studies, the association of low vitamin A from infrequent intake of fruits and vegetables with lung cancer risk has proved to be one of the more reproducible results achievable by epidemiologic methods. Willett (7) and Ziegler (8) have reviewed the results of many of these case-control investigations; they found that these several studies tend to demonstrate an approximate doubling of risk for the lowest level of dietary intake when compared with the highest. Willett has characterized the case-control studies as "remarkably consistent with the prospective studies in providing support for a protective relationship between carotenoid sources of vitamin A and occurrence of lung cancer" (7).

ESOPHAGEAL CANCER

No cancer shows greater variability in risk across populations than esophageal cancer. Populations in high-risk regions have rates 300 times greater than those in low-risk areas. Though many different factors have been studied and it seems likely that the disease has different etiologies in different regions, a common feature of many high-risk populations is poor diet. Several studies have examined the association of low fruit and vegetable consumption with esophageal cancer risk, and these have been reviewed recently by Graham and colleagues (9). Studies in China; Iran; Italy; Japan; Washington, DC; Buffalo, NY; and elsewhere have all shown a significantly increased risk associated with less frequent consumption of foods rich in β-carotene. Figure 2 shows the relationship between frequency of fruit and vegetable consumption and esophageal cancer risk as derived from a case-control investigation conducted at Roswell Park Memorial Institute (10).

The connection between esophageal cancer risk reduction and β-carotene intake is not as clear as it is for lung cancer. Exposure to ascorbic acid reportedly protects against gastric

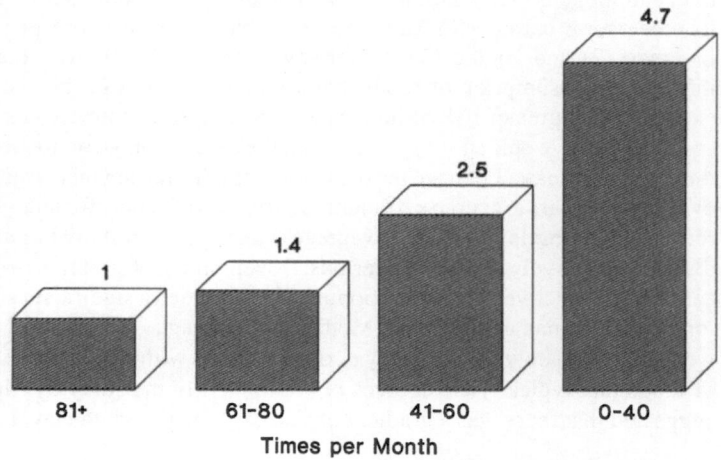

Figure 1. Relative risk associated with quintile level of reported β-carotene consumption by 569 lung cancer cases and 569 controls at Roswell Park Memorial Institute.

Times per Month

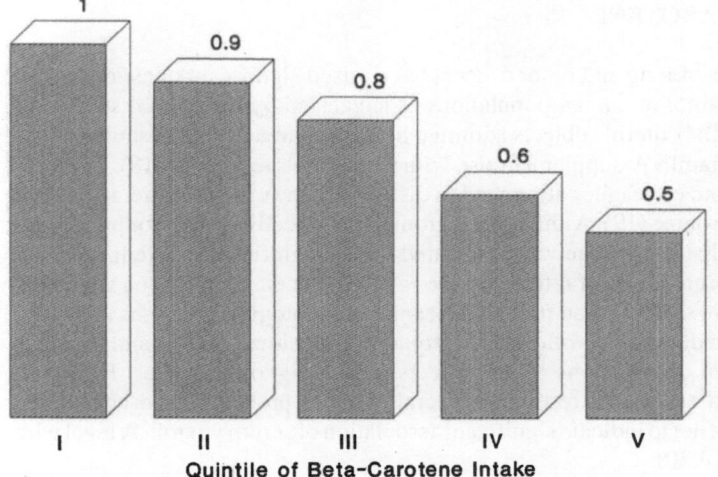

Figure 2. Relative risk for reported monthly frequency of vegetable and fruit consumption by 122 esophageal cancer cases and 235 controls at Roswell Park Memorial Institute.

Quintile of Beta-Carotene Intake

cancer, and it may serve the same role against esophageal cancer. Since many of the vegetables that are sources of β-carotene are also sources of vitamin C, distinguishing between β-carotene and vitamin C exposures is very difficult in observational studies. There also is little evidence that preformed dietary vitamin A acts as a protectant in the etiology of esophageal cancer. Graham and colleagues (9) examined dietary sources of retinol in a case-control study and found that increased consumption of such foods, principally meats and dairy products, was associated with increased, rather than decreased, risk for esophageal cancer.

ORAL AND LARYNGEAL CANCER

Though oral cancer in the United States is mainly the result of exposure to alcohol and tobacco, several studies have also linked low fruit and vegetable intake to increased risk for oral cancer. Winn and colleagues (11) found that females in their study who had oral cancer reported lower fruit and vegetable intake than control subjects. Marshall et al. found a dose-response relationship consistent with the hypothesis that foods rich in vitamin A reduce the risk of oral cancer (12). This relationship persisted even after control for the possible confounding roles of tobacco and alcohol. In India, where oral cancer is the most commonly occurring neoplasm, increased risk has been associated with lower fruit and vegetable intake. Serum studies also indicate that these types of patients have lower blood levels of β-carotene than controls (13). Furthermore, Stich and co-workers (14) demonstrated that administration of β-carotene decreased the frequency of micronucleated cells in the buccal mucosa of betel-nut and tobacco chewers in India, a group at high risk for oral cancer. These data may further suggest the protective potential of β-carotene exposure.

Risk for laryngeal cancer, like oral cancer, also appears to be affected by intake of fruits and vegetables rich in β-carotene. Graham and colleagues at Roswell Park Memorial Institute reported an increased risk of laryngeal cancer associated with infrequent consumption of foods that typically are sources of β-carotene (15). In a population-based study of the Texas Gulf Coast, Brown and colleagues found a significant tendency among laryngeal cancer patients to report less frequent fruit and vegetable consumption than controls (16). Similarly, a protective effect of diets rich in β-carotene was reported by La Vecchia and colleagues from a case-control study in Italy (17).

RETINOL VERSUS β-CAROTENE

Retrospective studies of lung and other cancers have raised significant questions about the protective effect of retinol in human populations as suggested by the animal studies. A survey of cancer patients and control subjects admitted to Boston-area hospitals showed little association of reported vitamin A-supplement use with cancer risk reduction (18). In a prospective study, Shekelle and colleagues attempted to distinguish the effects of dietary retinol from those of dietary β-carotene (19). Although they found no protective effect for preformed vitamin A, they did find that β-carotene was associated with a significant risk reduction.

The association of serum levels of retinol with long-term cancer risk has been studied in a number of cohorts. These studies often face significant methodologic challenges including issues of completeness and duration of follow-up, adequacy of specimen storage and analysis, and confounding of serum observations by the effects of prediagnostic cancer. However, different studies have had success in resolving several of these problems, and considered together, these studies tend not to indicate significant association of serum vitamin A level with subsequent cancer risk (7,8,20).

The relatively poor showing of retinol against β-carotene in epidemiologic studies of vitamin A and aerodigestive cancers in humans has significant potential implications for the future development of preventive interventions. These outcomes are not consistent with the demonstrated protective effects of preformed vitamin A in animal models and may suggest that these agents may not prove preferable as potential chemopreventive agents.

These epidemiologic outcomes may not, however, accurately reflect the relative importance of β-carotene and retinol in cancer prevention for several reasons. First, β-carotene intake may be more easily and accurately measured by epidemiologic questionnaires than preformed vitamin A. β-carotene is a relatively constant and stable nutrient in easily identified fruits and vegetables. Fat-soluble preformed vitamin A, on the other hand, occurs in variable amounts in dairy products, meats, and eggs; frequency of consumption of these foods may not be as good an indicator of vitamin A intake as frequency of fruit and vegetable consumption is of β-carotene intake. For instance, foods prepared with dairy products and eggs may contain "hidden" vitamin A of which the reporting subject is unaware. Vitamin A supplementation of foods is another factor confounding measurement. When using a food-frequency questionnaire, greater error in the measurement of preformed vitamin A than in that of β-carotene may occur; consequently, clearer findings for vitamin A than for β-carotene may result.

Second, it is also possible that the populations studied have been more homogeneous in exposure to preformed vitamin A than to its precursor β-carotene. Case-control and prospective research designs succeed only when variability in exposure is significant. In an intervention in which vitamin A exposure is manipulated to achieve this variability between study populations, the results that might be achieved may show different outcomes than a simple observational study. Finally, it is possible that the association of preformed vitamin A intake with risk reduction is confounded by its occurrence with other risk factors. For instance, high-fat diets that may have greater retinol content may have general effects that offset the possible benefit of the vitamin A. In contrast, diets high in β-carotene consumption derived from frequent fruit and vegetable intake may occur in the context of other risk-reducing aspects of life-style.

The strength and consistency of the epidemiologic findings concerning β-carotene and aerodigestive-cancer risk reduction compared with the weak and inconsistent effects found for preformed vitamin A may reflect the relative potential of these two dietary factors for preventing cancer. Such a conclusion, however, may test the limits of the power of epidemiologic methods alone to determine cancer-preventive effectiveness. In the case of preformed vitamin A, there may be more an absence of evidence of effect than evidence of an absence of effect. Clinical trials with preformed vitamin A and its synthetic analogues may therefore provide better evidence than observational epidemiology.

FUTURE RESEARCH

The question of the potential preventive power of preformed versus precursor vitamin A is only one of several questions about vitamin A and cancer that remain to be addressed. The epidemiologic data have mainly come from reports on the diets of persons relatively late in their lifespan or shortly prior to the onset of disease. Whether the period shortly prior to onset is the most important interval for the biologic effect of diet to be achieved is not determinable from the epidemiologic data. If it is, this would suggest that preventive interventions targeted to persons near the onset of disease can be effective. Alternatively, interventions will need to occur across a broader age range of the population. The question revolves around whether dietary sources of vitamin A act primarily as antipromoters or anti-initiators. Laboratory experimentation and clinical trial interventions will provide better data to address this timing of effects.

Another important issue concerns the relative potential of dietary and pharmacologic interventions. These two approaches offer different strengths and weaknesses. Dietary intervention may have low risk and a broad, sustained impact, but dietary preferences can be strongly held by those people whose resistance to change can be significant. Dietary interventions may also help reduce risk for heart disease and other conditions, in addition to cancer; however, dietary interventions are nonspecific, and many of the persons with other health problems to whom interventions are directed may not benefit from that intervention.

Chemopreventive strategies based on the use of pharmacologic agents such as vitamin A analogues have the advantage of permitting targeting of the intervention to persons in specific risk categories. If the numbers of persons who take vitamin supplements are any indication, chemoprevention may represent a change in life-style more easily adopted by persons at risk than dietary modification. Chemoprevention also has the advantage of achieving risk reduction in an individual more rapidly than dietary change.

CONCLUSION

The epidemiologic data, considered in aggregate, strongly indicate the likelihood that vitamin A exposure is associated with risk reduction for several types of aerodigestive cancer. In spite of the strength and consistency of the associations, however, epidemiologic data are limited in defining such relationships in detail. The mechanisms of action, the timing of effects, the optimal forms of intervention, and the actual benefit that may be achieved by intervention are all issues that go beyond current data. It may be that observational epidemiology has set the stage for the development of effective means of cancer prevention, but research in the laboratory, the clinic, and human populations is first required to establish the public-health significance of these observations.

REFERENCES

1. Sporn MB, Roberts AB. Role of retinoids in differentiation and carcinogenesis. Cancer Res 43:3034–3040, 1983.
2. Hirayama T. Diet and cancer. Nutr Cancer 1:67–81, 1979.
3. Bjelke E. Dietary vitamin A and human lung cancer. Int J Cancer 15:561–565, 1975.
4. MacLennan R, DaCosta J, Day NE, Law CH, Nq YK, Shanmugaratam K. Risk factors for lung cancer in Singapore Chinese. Int J Cancer 20:854–860, 1977.
5. Mettlin C, Graham S, Swanson M. Vitamin A and lung cancer. J Natl Cancer Inst 62:1435–1438, 1979.
6. Mettlin C. Milk drinking, other beverage habits and lung cancer risk. Int J Cancer 43:608–612, 1989.
7. Willett WC. Vitamin A and lung cancer. Nutr Rev 48:201–211, 1990.
8. Ziegler RG. A review of epidemiologic evidence that carotenoids reduce the risk of cancer. J Nutr 119:116–122, 1989.

9. Graham S, Marshall J, Haughey B, Brasure J, Fruedenheim J, Ziclezny M, Wilkinson G, Nolan J. Nutritional epidemiology of cancer of the esophagus. Am J Epidemiol 131:454–467, 1990.

10. Mettlin C, Graham S, Priore R, Marshall J, Swanson M. Diet and cancer of the esophagus. Nutr Cancer 2:143–147, 1981.

11. Winn DM, Ziegler RG, Pickle LW. Diet in the etiology of oral and pharyngeal cancer among women from the southern United States. Cancer Res 44:1216–1222, 1984.

12. Marshall J, Graham S, Mettlin C, Shedd D, Swanson M. Diet in the epidemiology of oral cancer. Nutr Cancer 3:145–149, 1981.

13. Notani PN, Sanghvi LD. Role of diet in cancers of the oral cavity. Indian J Cancer 13:156–160, 1976.

14. Stich HF, Stich W, Rosin MP, Vallejera WO. Use of the micronucleus test to monitor the effect of vitamin A, beta-carotene, and canthaxanthin on the buccal mucosa of betel nut/tobacco chewers. Int J Cancer 34:745–750,1984.

15. Graham S, Mettlin C, Marshall J, Priore R, Rzepka T, Shedd D. Dietary factors in the epidemiology of cancer of the larynx. Am J Epidemiol 113:675–680, 1981.

16. Brown LM, Mason TJ, Pickle LW, Stewart PA, Buffler PA, Burau K, Ziegler RG, Fraumeni JF. Occupational risk factors for laryngeal cancer on the Texas Gulf Coast. Cancer Res 48:1960–1964, 1988.

17. La Vecchia C, Negri E, D'Avanzo B, Franceschi S, Decarli A, Boyle P. Dietary indicators of laryngeal cancer risk. Cancer Res 50:4497–4500, 1990.

18. Smith PG, Jick H. Cancers among users of preparations containing vitamin A. Cancer 42:808–811, 1978.

19. Shekelle RB, Lepper M, Liu S, Maliza C, Raynor WJ Jr, Rossof AH, Paul O, Stamler J. Dietary vitamin A and risk of cancer in the Western Electric study. Lancet 2:1185–1190, 1981.

20. Hennekens CH. Vitamin A analogues in cancer chemoprevention. In DeVita VT Jr, Hellman S, Rosenberg SA (eds): Important Advances in Oncology. Philadelphia: JB Lippincott, 1986, pp. 23–35.

Multiple Primary Squamous Carcinomas of the Upper Aerodigestive Tract

Robert M. Byers

Department of Head and Neck Surgery
The University of Texas M. D. Anderson Cancer Center
Houston, Texas

INTRODUCTION

Thirty to 40,000 patients develop cancer of the upper aerodigestive tract each year. This group comprises approximately 5% of all cancers. The most common type is squamous carcinoma, arising in the mucous membranes of the larynx, hypopharynx, oropharynx, nasopharynx, and oral cavity. Survival after treatment for these cancers is usually very poor, but not necessarily because of recurrent disease. These patients are of advanced age with poor nutrition and many associated medical problems that adversely affect the patient's longevity. In addition, because most of these patients have mucosal changes throughout their entire upper aerodigestive tract, "a field of cancerization," they are at risk for the development of second carcinomas (1). The survival of approximately one third of these patients is a direct result of the biologic behavior of a second synchronous or metachronous primary cancer (2–4). The type of treatment given for the initial or "index" cancer has a major effect on how the second cancer is treated. There is no evidence that the use of radiation can prevent this phenomenon and, in fact, its previous use may compromise the ideal treatment for the subsequent cancer (5). Almost every paper published today dealing with the treatment of squamous carcinomas of the head and neck ends commenting on "the survival of patients with head and neck squamous carcinomas will not be markedly improved until the question of second cancers in the upper aerodigestive tract is addressed." In any list of reasons for failure of treatment of a squamous carcinoma of the head and neck, the following are considered: local regional failure, distant metastasis, complications of treatment, intercurrent disease, and *second primary cancers*. The problem with second primary cancers has been around a long time and, in fact, in an autopsy series in 1932 that consisted of 1078 examinations of cancer patients, multiple cancers were found in 40, which represented 3.7% (6).

The definition of a second primary cancer depends on several factors, such as 1) any cancer of a different histology; 2) any cancer of the same histology, but separated geographically by at least 2 cm from the first; and 3) any cancer occurring at least 3 years after the first cancer. If the new cancer is in the lung, it must be histologically different from the initial cancer, unless it occurs 3 or more years later (6). Synchronous primary cancers are those that develop within 6 months of the index cancer, and metachronous cancers are those that develop after 6 months.

The Biology and Prevention of Aerodigestive Tract Cancers
Edited by G.R.Newell and W.K. Hong, Plenum Press, New York, 1992

CLINICAL STUDIES

The use of triple endoscopy has been proposed as a means for early detection of synchronous or metachronous cancers. This involves an invasive procedure consisting of laryngoscopy, bronchoscopy, and esophagoscopy. The usual cost to the patient can range from $1000 to $2500. In the series published in 1982, Dr. A. Weaver presented 271 patients with biopsy-proven head and neck squamous carcinoma who were evaluated with triple endoscopy (7). Sixty-nine (25%) had had at least one other primary tumor in either the head and neck, lung, or the esophagus identified on the initial examination (10%) or subsequent follow-up (15%). Twenty-eight patients (10%) had synchronous cancers of which 13 (49%) were in the head and neck. Eleven had head and neck plus esophageal cancers, two had head and neck plus lung cancer, and two had head and neck plus lung and esophageal cancers. Of the entire group of 271 patients, only 5.5% of the second cancers would have been picked up by bronchoscopy and/or esophagoscopy. More important, however, only 1.5% of these patients were asymptomatic. The cost-benefit ratio with this procedure is questionable.

Dr. S. Strong reported a series of 100 patients with biopsy-proven squamous carcinoma of the upper aerodigestive tract who smoked more than two packs of cigarettes per day. All of these patients had biopsies of normal-appearing oral mucosa, and all but one had electron microscopy abnormalities suggestive of premalignant changes. During the follow-up period for these 100 patients, 26 developed second cancers within 3 years (8).

In a study of 2151 patients with primary head and neck cancers treated with surgery, radiation, or both, and followed from 5 to 30 years, 178 developed second cancers of which 39 arose in the head and neck. There was no statistical difference in the development of the second head and neck cancers with either modality of treatment or in the time to develop the second head and neck cancer. However, the type of treatment for the index cancer obviously did affect how the second cancer was treated (9).

In a study of 351 patients with cancer of the oral tongue, the incidence of second cancers with a 5–20-year follow-up was 27% for those who used tobacco and alcohol. Seventy-three percent of these patients died of their second cancer. In this same group of 351 patients, 18.5% who did not use tobacco or alcohol developed a second cancer, and 60% of these patients died of the second cancer (10).

In a series of 3490 patients with cancer of the oral cavity, 59 presented with two or more synchronous cancers of which 2% were in the head and neck region. Sixty-one patients developed metachronous cancers that represented, again, approximately 2% of the entire group (11).

In a series of 384 patients with oropharynx cancer seen between 1964 and 1968 and followed for at least 5 years or more, 54 (37%) developed a second cancer in the embryonic foregut. Half of these cancers developed in patients with Tl-T2 N0 index cancers. The sites of the second cancers were oral cavity, hypopharynx, esophagus, and lung. Thirty-six (66%) died as a result of this second cancer.

The development of esophageal cancer has been associated with patients who have primary cancers in the supraglottic larynx and oropharynx, whereas patients with glottic cancers develop, more often, second cancers in the lung (12). The amount of smoking prior to development of the index primary or after treatment for the index primary seems to affect the timing in the development of the second cancer. Although not statistically significant, patients who smoked the greatest amount developed a second cancer in less than 5 years after the first, while patients who smoked the least went 10 years or more before developing a second cancer. This was true even if the heaviest smokers gave up smoking when they developed the first cancer (13).

CONCLUSION

In summary, the patient with the diagnosis of squamous carcinoma of the upper aerodigestive tract is in double jeopardy. The longer he lives following treatment of his initial or index cancer, the greater the likelihood he has of developing a second cancer in either the head and neck, esophagus, or the lung. Even if he discontinues the use of tobacco products and alcohol, he still runs a significant risk. Aggressive measures to prevent this phenomenon are certainly desirable from the standpoint of the individual patient and society in general (14). The economic consequences are enormous.

REFERENCES

1. Slaughter DP, Southwick HW, Smejkal W. "Field cancerization" in oral stratified squamous epithelium: Clinical implications of multicentric origin. Cancer 6:963–968, 1953.
2. Lippman SM, Ang WK. Second malignant tumors in head and neck squamous cell carcinoma: The overshadowing threat for patients with early-stage disease. Int J Radiat Oncol Biol Phys 17:691–694, 1989.
3. Licciardello JT, Spitz MR, Hong WK. Multiple primary cancer in patients with cancer of the head and neck: Second cancer of the head and neck, esophagus, and lung. Int J Radiat Oncol Biol Phys 17:467–476, 1989.
4. Jesse RH, Sugarbaker EV. Squamous cell carcinoma of the oropharynx: Why we fail. Am J Surg 132:435–438, 1976.
5. Cooper JS, Pajak TF, Rubin P, Tupchong L, Brady LW, Leibel SA, Laramore GE, Marcial VA, Davis LW, Cox JD. Second malignancies in patients who have head and neck cancer: Incidence, effect on survival and implications based on the RTOG experience. Int J Radiat Oncol Biol Phys 17:449–456, 1989.
6. Warren S, Gates O. Multiple primary malignant tumors. A survey of the literature and a statistical study. Am J Cancer 16:1358–1414, 1932.
7. Atkinson D, Fleming S, Weaver A. Triple endoscopy: A valuable procedure in head and neck surgery. Am J Surg 144:416–420, 1982.
8. Incze J, Vaughan C, Leu P, Strong S, Kulapaditharom B. Premalignant changes in normal appearing epithelium in patients with squamous cell carcinoma of the upper aerodigestive tract. Am J Surg 144:401–406, 1982.
9. Parker RG, Enstrom JE. Second primary cancers of the head and neck following treatment of initial primary head and neck cancers. Int J Radiat Oncol Biol Phys 14:561–564, 1986.
10. Johnston WD, Ballantyne AJ. Prognostic effect of tobacco and alcohol use in patients with oral tongue cancer. Am J Surg 134:444–447, 1977.
11. MacComb W, Fletcher G. Cancer of the Head and Neck. Baltimore: Williams & Wilkins, 1957, pp. 21.
12. McDonald S, Haie C, Rubin P, Nelson D, Divers LD. Second malignant tumors in patients with laryngeal carcinoma: Diagnosis, treatment, and prevention. Int J Radiat Oncol Biol Phys 17:457–465, 1989.
13. Wynder EL, Dodo H, Bloch DA, Gantt RC, Moore OS. Epidemiologic investigation of multiple primary cancer of the upper alimentary and respiratory tracts. Cancer 4:730–739, 1969.
14. Hong WK, Lippman SM, Itri LM, Karp DD, Lee JS, Byers RM, Schantz SP, Kramer AM, Lotan R, Peters LJ, Dimery IW, Brown BW, Goepfert H. Prevention of second primary tumors with isotretinoin in squamous cell carcinoma of the head and neck. N Engl J Med 323:795–801, 1990.

Genetic and Environmental Interactions as Risks for Aerodigestive Cancers

Margaret R. Spitz,[1] T. C. Hsu,[2] and Stimson P. Schantz[3]

[1]Department of Cancer Prevention and Control
[2]Department of Cell Biology
The University of Texas M. D. Anderson Cancer Center
Houston, Texas

[3]Department of Head and Neck Surgery
Memorial Sloan-Kettering Cancer Center
New York, New York

INTRODUCTION

Only a fraction of people exposed to carcinogens will ultimately develop cancer. This fact suggests that individuals are unique with respect to cancer risk and that in the general population, there is a broad range of susceptibility to carcinogenesis. These variations in susceptibility as well as in cancer incidence in different ethnic groups may be genetically determined, at least in part. The study of genetic susceptibility and exogenous carcinogens—their relationship and interaction—is the basis for the important emerging science of ecogenetics.

Ecogenetics is the study of genetic and environmental relationships and interactions using analytic epidemiologic techniques. It is a science that fosters interdisciplinary collaborative research and is of special relevance to carcinogenesis, in which genetic susceptibility may determine the ultimate host response to exogenous exposures.

Based on available epidemiologic data, up to 90% of the cancer present in the U.S. population can be attributed to life-style and other environmental factors (1). These estimates, however, obscure significant intraindividual variability in other factors that modify carcinogenesis, the binding of drugs and carcinogens, and DNA repair capability (2). The identification of markers such as these may ultimately have a positive impact on cancer prevention and control. The information that follows will focus on one such marker of susceptibility to cancer risk, DNA repair capability.

DNA REPAIR CAPABILITY

If permanent genetic damage is to be avoided, the active metabolites of a particular carcinogen that has bound to DNA must be removed by enzymatic repair mechanisms (3). Hsu has hypothesized that within the general population there is a spectrum of DNA repair

The Biology and Prevention of Aerodigestive Tract Cancers
Edited by G.R.Newell and W.K. Hong, Plenum Press, New York, 1992

31

capability (4). At one end of the spectrum are people with chromosome breakage syndromes characterized by high numbers of spontaneous chromosome breaks, unusual susceptibility to induction of breaks by clastogens, and increased cancer risks. Evidence for a DNA repair deficiency within this group is also strong in xeroderma pigmentosum, in which patients show susceptibility to sunlight-induced skin damage and a heightened risk for cutaneous tumors, though not an increased frequency of spontaneous chromosome aberrations.

Even within the general asymptomatic population, there may be varying degrees of repair capability. Hsu hypothesized that people with mild degrees of mutagen sensitivity may be more likely than those without the sensitivity to accumulate mutations and chromosome aberrations in their cells and thus may become more susceptible to the initiation of cancer (5).

EXPERIMENTAL PROTOCOL

Hsu has developed a list assay to demonstrate this variation in repair capability, a latent genetic instability. As an indicator of mutagen susceptibility, Hsu's assay quantifies the chromosome breaks induced in vitro by bleomycin in short-term, cultured lymphocytes (6). Bleomycin is a radiomimetic drug that induces single- and double-stranded DNA breaks.

For the test, a peripheral blood sample (10 ml or less) is collected from each donor in a heparinized tube and stored at 4°C. The standard blood culture procedure uses RPMI-1640 medium, supplemented with 20% fetal calf serum and phytohemagglutinin, in a 1:9 ratio of blood to medium. After 67 hours of incubation, one set of cultures is treated for 5 hours with bleomycin (0.03 μg/ml). Colcemid (demecolcine) (0.04 μg/ml) is added in the last hour to induce mitotic arrest prior to harvesting. A conventional cell-harvesting procedure follows. The cells are treated with hypotonic KCl (0.07 M) solution for 15–20 minutes, fixed, washed with a freshly prepared 3:1 mixture of methanol and acetic acid, and air-dried on wet slides. The slides are then stained with Giemsa solution without banding. Fifty well-spread metaphases are examined from coded slides. The chromatid aberrations recorded are either frank chromatid breaks or exchanges. Bleomycin tends to induce few chromatid exchanges (which, if present, are considered as two breaks). Chromatid gaps and attenuated regions are disregarded. The frequency of breakage is expressed as breaks per cell (b/c) for purposes of comparison.

ANALYSES OF MUTAGEN SENSITIVITY

In Cancer Patients

Our first objective was to evaluate the role of mutagen sensitivity as a risk factor for upper aerodigestive tract cancer. We compared mutagen sensitivity to bleomycin-induced chromosome damage in 75 patients (53 men and 22 women) with previously untreated, upper aerodigestive tract malignancies with sensitivity in 62 healthy control subjects selected from among hospital employees (7). Data on tobacco and alcohol use were derived from detailed, self-administered cancer risk factor questionnaires, which The University of Texas M. D. Anderson Cancer Center (Houston, TX) distributes to all newly registered adult patients (8).

Baseline mutagen sensitivity values were established on the patients and the controls. Forty-five patients and 13 controls were sensitive to bleomycin-induced mutagenesis (average b/c > 0.8). Differential susceptibility was detected in patients categorized by primary tumor location. Odds ratios (OR) for chromosome sensitivity were significantly elevated for all sites (OR = 10.3 for pharyngeal cancers, 8.0 for laryngeal cancers, and 3.8 for oral cavity cancers). On logistic regression analysis, mutagen sensitivity remained a strong and independent risk factor after adjustment for potential confounding from age, sex, and use of tobacco and alcohol (OR = 4.3; 95% confidence limits = 2.0, 10.2).

To evaluate the independent effect of chromosome sensitivity as well as the interaction of chromosome sensitivity with cigarette smoking and alcohol consumption, risk estimates for various combinations of sensitivity and either smoking or alcohol use were computed in stratified analyses. These analyses were restricted to study participants for whom all relevant information was available. Referent categories were study participants who were not mutagen sensitive and who used neither cigarettes nor alcohol. The data were sparse in some categories, and the resultant measures of effect were therefore somewhat unstable. Mutagen sensitivity was a risk factor in the absence of smoking (OR = 5.8) and of alcohol use (OR = 3.6), and there were significantly elevated risks associated with either smoking or alcohol use in chromosome-stable persons (OR = 5.4 in each instance). The combined effects of chromosome sensitivity and either smoking (OR = 19.8) or alcohol use (OR = 17.1) were consistent with a multiplicative scale of no interaction.

In Cigarette Smokers

Because of the relationship between cigarette smoking and aerodigestive cancers, an attempt was made to measure the bleomycin sensitivity of asymptomatic individuals who had long smoking histories (4). For the hypothesis to be valid, there would have been a higher proportion of less sensitive individuals among the older smokers. In fact, the bleomycin-sensitivity profile of older smokers (older than 50) with a 20-year smoking history and no history of cancer placed only 1.78% of the subjects in the hypersensitive class (b/c > 1.0). These data suggest that older smokers represent the bleomycin-resistant subpopulation of the control population, perhaps because the sensitive subpopulation had already developed lung cancer or another smoking-related malignancy. This finding contrasted sharply with the observation that there was no significant difference between the sensitivity profiles of younger smokers and normal controls (25% mutagen sensitive) and suggested that there are no immediate shifts in bleomycin sensitivity which are due merely to smoking itself.

MUTAGEN SENSITIVITY AS A PREDICTOR OF RISK

Our next focus was to evaluate the usefulness of mutagen sensitivity as a predictor of cancer risk. Patients with upper aerodigestive tract cancers are at a high risk for the development of second malignant tumors, especially in tobacco-exposed tissues. These patients are thus ideally suited for prospective analysis.

Eighty-four patients with previously untreated aerodigestive tract cancers received a baseline assessment for mutagen sensitivity and self-reported life-style exposures (9). Sixty-two of these patients had been included in the previous case-control study (7). After surgery or radiotherapy, or both, they were followed up longitudinally (median time = 20 mo, range 4–31 mo) for the development of second malignancies. Histologically confirmed multiple primary malignancies were defined by criteria established in 1932 by Warren and Gates (10).

Of the 33 hypersensitive patients, nine (27%) developed subsequent primary cancers, compared with only four (8%) of the 51 mutagen-stable patients (OR = 4.4; confidence limits = 1.2, 15.8). There were no substantive differences between mutagen-sensitive and mutagen-stable patients with regard to age, sex, treatment modality, or use of tobacco or alcohol.

Predictably, patients who developed second malignant tumors had a more extensive smoking history than did those who did not, although these differences were not statistically significant. Logistic regression analysis of multiple primary cancer risks independent of any categorical grouping showed a significant relationship between an increasing risk of multiple primaries and an incrementally increasing mutagen-sensitivity value ($P = 0.02$). Despite the small study size and the short period of follow-up evaluation, the data support the hypothesis that mutagen-sensitive patients constitute a target subpopulation for careful scrutiny. Thus, the identification of high-risk subpopulations has both clinical and prognostic relevance.

CONCLUSION

The use of genetic markers clearly enhances the power and precision of epidemiologic research. The preventive implications of precise and valid markers for carcinogen sensitivity are clear. We are aware of the need for extensive validation of the assay and for rigorously designed and conducted epidemiologic studies. Nevertheless, the strength of the association between cancer risk and mutagen sensitivity is impressive, despite the inherent problems in the size and design of the studies. The thesis that chromosome instability and defective DNA repair may underlie susceptibility to environmental carcinogenesis is plausible and presents a promising avenue for further research.

REFERENCES

1. Doll R, Peto R. The causes of cancer: Quantitative estimates of avoidable risk of cancer in the United States today. London: Oxford University Press, 1981.
2. Perera F, Boffetta P. Perspectives on comparing risks of environmental carcinogens. J Natl Cancer Inst 80:1282–1293, 1988.
3. Vahakangas K, Pelkonen O. Host variation in carcinogen metabolism and DNA repair. In Lynch HT, Hirayama T (eds): Genetic Epidemiology of Cancer. Florida: CRC Press, 1989, pp. 35–54.
4. Hsu TC, Johnston DA, Cherry LM, Ramkissoon D, Schantz SP, Jessup JM, Winn R, Shirley L, Furlong C. Sensitivity to genotoxic effects of bleomycin in humans: Possible relationship to environmental carcinogenesis. Int J Cancer 43:403–409, 1989.
5. Hsu TC. Genetic predisposition to cancer with special reference to mutagen sensitivity. In-Vitro Cell Dev Biol 23:591–603, 1987.
6. Cherry LM, Hsu TC. Bleomycin-induced chromosome damage in lymphocytes of medullary thyroid carcinoma patients and their family members. Anticancer Res 3:367–372, 1983.
7. Spitz MR, Fueger JJ, Beddingfield NA, Annegers JF, Hsu TC, Newell GR, Schantz SP. Chromosome sensitivity to bleomycin-induced mutagenesis: An independent risk factor for upper aerodigestive tract cancers. Cancer Res 49:4626–4628, 1989.
8. Spitz MR, Fueger JJ, Borrud LG, Newell GR. The development of a comprehensive, institutional-based patient risk evaluation program: I. Development, content, and data management. Am J Prev Med 4:183–187, 1988.
9. Schantz SP, Spitz MR, Hsu TC. Mutagen sensitivity in patients with head and neck cancers: A biologic marker for risk of multiple primary malignancies. J Natl Cancer Inst 82:1773–1775, 1990.
10. Warren S, Gates O. Multiple primary malignant tumors: A survey of the literature and a statistical study. American Journal of Cancer 16:1358–1414, 1932.

Alcohol: A Cocarcinogen in Head and Neck Malignancies

T. C. Hsu

Department of Cell Biology
The University of Texas M. D. Anderson Cancer Center
Houston, Texas

Most geneticists and biochemists who work on environmental mutagenesis agree that environmental carcinogenesis is caused by agents that induce genotoxicity, including mutations, chromosome aberrations, and mitotic anomalies, in somatic cells. However, not every person develops cancer after similar exposure to mutagens, such as tobacco. It is generally believed that sensitivity to mutagens, hence susceptibility to cancer, is a reflection of a person's innate capability to repair genetic damage (of DNA and chromosomes) inflicted by mutagens.

Studies of several chromosome instability syndromes, all of which are rare maladies, have shed much light on the problem relating to genetic disturbances and the resulting propensity toward neoplastic initiation (1). The clinical and genetic pictures of two of these syndromes, xeroderma pigmentosum and Bloom's syndrome, are especially enlightening because they clearly indicate the relationship between repair deficiency and cancer susceptibility. Patients with xeroderma pigmentosum lack the repair mechanism by which damaged DNA segments (pyrimidine dimers) induced by ultraviolet light are cleaved (2–4); consequently, these patients are highly susceptible to cutaneous malignancies following exposure to sunlight. The genetic defect of Bloom's syndrome is a deficiency in DNA ligase I (5,6); thus, these patients are not able to repair spontaneous chromosome breakages effectively, and genetic damage accumulates.

Paradoxically, alcohol acting alone has been regarded as a cancer risk of the upper aerodigestive tract (7,8). Numerous investigations, employing a variety of test materials and test protocols, have shown that ethyl alcohol is not a mutagen until it is metabolically converted by alcohol dehydrogenase into acetaldehyde, which is a mutagen (9). Since there is no evidence for an abnormally high activity of alcohol dehydrogenase in the epithelial cells of the oral cavity, the larynx, or the pharynx, the role of alcohol in carcinogenesis of the upper aerodigestive tract remains to be elucidated. Several hypotheses have been proposed: (a) Minute quantities of carcinogens found in some brands of beer and Scotch whiskey may be the cause; (b) alcohol may increase the solubility of contaminating carcinogens that find their way into the oral cavity; and (c) alcohol may increase the permeability of the epithelial cells. But these and other possible interpretations lack support by experimental data.

The Biology and Prevention of Aerodigestive Tract Cancers
Edited by G.R.Newell and W.K. Hong, Plenum Press, New York, 1992

In a recent editorial (10), the author considered alcohol as a cocarcinogen, implying that a nonmutagen, such as alcohol, may enhance the genotoxic potential of a particular carcinogen when the two substances interact. If this indeed is the case, then ethyl alcohol richly deserves the term cocarcinogen; for, as two teams of investigators independently discovered, when cultured mammalian cells were exposed simultaneously to mutagens and ethanol, the frequencies of chromosome damage increased, compared with those exposed to mutagens alone (8,11). This synergistic effect with alcohol was found to be dose dependent; that is, lower concentrations of alcohol (0.5% or lower) were not effective, but with higher concentrations (1% or above), the increase of chromosome breakage was dramatic. Moreover, this synergistic effect was not limited to one type of mutagen. Mutagens with different genotoxic mechanisms showed similar responses when they were applied in conjunction with ethanol. It appears, therefore, that the synergism does not result from the formation of a compound molecule that has more genotoxic potential than the original mutagen molecule; rather, it may be the result of a more general process related to the alcohol.

Our study examined the possibility that ethanol at high concentrations interferes with DNA repair. DNA repair is a capability most people possess (except those few who may lack a particular DNA repair enzyme). This repair phenomenon was described decades ago. Cytogeneticists working on radiation-induced chromosome damage demonstrated that rates of chromosome aberrations were inversely related to the time lapse between irradiation and cell harvest.

To investigate our hypothesis that alcohol can inhibit or retard DNA repair, we designed a test protocol using pulse treatments. Continuous cotreatment, the routine experimental protocol, was not suitable because with this type of treatment, the repair of chromatid breaks and the generation of new chromatid breaks occur simultaneously. Under such conditions, it is not possible to calculate repair kinetics.

We treated cell populations with bleomycin for 10 minutes, washing off the mutagen as thoroughly as possible and reincubating the cells in three different media: a control growth medium, a medium with 0.5% ethanol, and a medium with 2% ethanol. The cultures were harvested 1, 3, and 5 hours after the removal of the bleomycin. When the cells were reincubated in the control medium and in the medium with 0.5% alcohol, clear evidence for repair was recorded for all cell lines tested, including those derived from patients with ataxia-telangiectasia, who are known to be radiosensitive and bleomycin-sensitive. Conversely, when cells were reincubated in the medium containing 2% alcohol, there was no reduction of chromatid breakage rates in any of the samples. These data (12) strongly indicate that ethyl alcohol, at concentrations of 2% or higher, inhibits cellular DNA repair, at least as long as the ethanol is present.

The overwhelming majority of chemical carcinogens in air, water, and food enter the body through the upper aerodigestive tract. These contaminants, not to mention tobacco smoke, can induce mutations and chromosome breakage in the cells of epithelial tissue, but presumably most lesions are removed by various repair enzymes. When alcoholic beverages are consumed, however, DNA repair ceases temporarily, and a number of genetic lesions continue to form; thus the mutation load may accumulate. If alcohol at a concentration of just 2% can stop DNA repair, then the potentially devastating effect becomes apparent for all alcoholic beverages, ranging from 5% ethyl alcohol for wine coolers to 50% for whiskey. Moreover, whereas alcohol becomes substantially diluted during its journey through the body and thus affects the cells of internal organs with decreasing intensity, it makes contact with the epithelial cells of the oral cavity at full strength. Therefore, when alcohol consumption is combined with cancer-causing activities like cigarette smoking and betel nut chewing, the risk of cancer of the upper digestive tract increases dramatically.

REFERENCES

1. German J. Chromosome Mutation and Neoplasia. New York: Alan R Liss, 1983.
2. Setlow RB, Regan JD, German J, Carrier WL. Evidence that xeroderma pigmentosum cells do not perform the first step in the repair of ultra-violet damage to DNA. Proc Natl Acad Sci USA 64:1035–1041, 1969.
3. Cleaver J, Bootsma D. Xeroderma pigmentosum: Biochemical and genetic characteristics. Annual Review of Genetics 9:19–38, 1975.
4. Parrington JM, Delhanty JDA, Baden HP. Unscheduled DNA synthesis, UV-induced chromosome aberrations and SV40 transformation in cultured cells from xeroderma pigmentosum. Ann Hum Genet 35:149–160, 1971.
5. Willis AE, Weksberg R, Tomlinson S, Lindhahl T. Structural alterations of DNA ligase I in Bloom syndrome. Proc Natl Acad Sci USA 84:8016–8020, 1987.
6. Chan JYH, Becker FF, German J, Ray JH. Altered DNA ligase I activity in Bloom's syndrome cells. Nature 325:357–359, 1987.
7. Spitz MR, Fueger JJ, Beddingfield NA, Annegers JF, Hsu TC, Newell GR, Schantz SP. Chromosome sensitivity to bleomycin-induced mutagenesis, an independent risk factor for upper aerodigestive tract cancers. Cancer Res 49:4626–4628, 1989.
8. Hsu TC, Furlong C, Spitz MR. Ethyl alcohol as a cocarcinogen with special reference to the aerodigestive tract: A cytogenetic study. Anticancer Res, in press.
9. Obe G, Anderson D. Genetic effects of ethanol. Mutat Res 186:177–200, 1987.
10. Editorial: Alcohol and cancer. Lancet 1:634–635, 1990.
11. Lin YC, Ho IC, Lee TC. Ethanol and acetaldehyde potentiate the clastogenicity of ultraviolet light, methyl methane-sulfonate, mitomycin C and bleomycin in Chinese hamster ovary cells. Mutat Res 216:93–99, 1989.
12. Hsu TC, Furlong C. Anticancer Res, in press.

Smokeless Tobacco and Aerodigestive Tract Cancers: Recent Research Directions

Deborah M. Winn

National Center for Health Statistics
Centers for Disease Control
Hyattsville, Maryland

INTRODUCTION

Though smokeless tobacco, which includes chewing tobacco and snuff, was the most common form of tobacco used at the turn of the century (1), its use declined over subsequent decades. In the mid-1970s, however, its popularity again rose, leading to a 56% increase in snuff use from 1970 to 1985, accounted for by moist snuff, and a 36% increase in chewing tobacco, attributed to loose-leaf tobacco (2). With the exception of a leveling off around 1987, this upward trend in use has continued (3).

Recognition of smokeless tobacco as a new (or more precisely, a recurring) public health problem came in the early 1980s, partly as a result of concern over the renewed popularity of these products. Simultaneously with the rise in use, research on two major fronts—epidemiologic investigations and laboratory work on carcinogenesis—yielded much information about the carcinogenic potential of smokeless tobacco. Also during the early 1980s, there was an increasing awareness that high mortality rates of oral cancer resulting from use of American or European unsmoked tobaccos had clear parallels with the high rates of smokeless tobacco–caused aerodigestive tract cancers among many cultures throughout the world.

One epidemiologic study published in 1981 provided strong evidence of a strong relationship between snuff use and oral and pharynx cancer (4) among women in North Carolina. In that study, women using snuff were estimated to quadruple their risk of oral and pharynx cancer. For cancers of the buccal mucosa and gums, the risks were dramatically higher. These findings explained the epidemic of oral cancer mortality among women observed in cancer maps covering the period 1950–1969 (5), which was one of the reasons for initiating the study. These findings also were consistent with numerous case reports in the literature documenting oral cancer in long-term users of smokeless tobacco (6). Other case-control studies provided additional support to the evidence for smokeless tobacco as a cause of oral cancer, since consistently strong associations were observed and confounding influences of other risk factors such as smoking could be ruled out in some studies (2). Smokeless tobacco use also seems to be linked to other upper aerodigestive cancer sites (i.e., the larynx and the esophagus [2]), although evidence does not appear sufficiently extensive at this time to label smokeless tobacco as a cause of these cancers. Some positive findings have been observed for other cancer sites, but the evidence is either inconclusive or inconsistent. Smokeless tobacco seems not to be a risk factor for bladder cancer (2).

The Biology and Prevention of Aerodigestive Tract Cancers
Edited by G.R.Newell and W.K. Hong, Plenum Press, New York, 1992

Simultaneously with the epidemiologic work, experimental and laboratory studies of the carcinogenicity of smokeless tobaccos were under way. This work led to an understanding of the basis for the carcinogenicity of snuff and chewing tobacco. Smokeless tobaccos contain tobacco-specific N-nitrosamines, which have been shown to cause cancer in laboratory animals. These tobacco-specific nitrosamines occur in high amounts in smokeless tobacco, several orders of magnitude higher than in other consumer products (7). Two of the most important N-nitrosamines are N-nitrosonornicotine (NNN) and 4-(N-methyl-N-nitrosamino)-1-(3-pyridyl)-1-butanone (NNK). Other carcinogenic substances in small amounts in smokeless tobacco include polonium 210 and benzo[a]pyrene (8).

As a result of this new information, the mid-1980s saw considerable public attention and public policy focused on the problem of smokeless tobacco and cancer. A number of major scientific bodies evaluated the world literature and labeled smokeless tobacco or snuff as a cause of oral cancer, including an advisory group to the U.S. Surgeon General (2), the International Agency for Research on Cancer (6), a National Institutes of Health Consensus Conference (9), and others. In 1986, the U.S. Congress banned electronic advertising of smokeless tobacco products and decreed that warning labels be included on packages of smokeless tobacco (10). Work on the carcinogenicity of smokeless tobacco has continued since the mid-1980s into the 1990s; these recent efforts are described in this report.

RECENT EPIDEMIOLOGIC STUDIES OF SMOKELESS TOBACCO AND CANCER

As shown in the table, three recent epidemiologic studies published from 1986 to 1988 have examined the relationship between smokeless tobacco and oral cancer risk.

In the first study, researchers at The University of Texas M. D. Anderson Cancer Center (Houston, TX) analyzed 185 patients with upper aerodigestive tract cancers (oral cavity, oropharynx, larynx, and tongue) seen from 1985 through February 1987 and compared them with an equal number of controls with cancers that were not squamous cell carcinomas (11). Snuff use was associated with an elevated risk for these cancers based on nine cases and four controls (odds ratio, 3.4; 95% confidence interval, 1.0–10.9). However, it was noted that all of the nine cases and three of the four controls smoked, making it impossible to evaluate the independent influences of these habits. Equal numbers of case and control patients used chewing tobacco.

A large case-control study of head and neck cancers was undertaken using the Florida Cancer Data System, which collects data on all cancer patients in the state (12). Most of the

Table. Recent Case-Control Studies of Smokeless Tobacco and Oral/Pharynx Cancer

Data Source	Cancer Site for Cases	Relative Risk and 95% Confidence Limits for Users
Florida Cancer Data System (Stockwell, Lyman, 1986)	Tongue	2.3 (0.2–12.9)[a]
	Mouth/gum	11.2 (4.1–30.7)[a]
	Pharynx	4.1 (0.9–18.0)[a]
Four U.S. cancer registries (Blot et al., 1988)	Mouth, pharynx	6.2 (1.9–19.8)[b]
M. D. Anderson Cancer Center, Houston, TX (Spitz et al., 1988)	Mouth, pharynx, larynx	3.4 (1.0–10.9)[c]

[a]Controlling for age, race, sex, and smoking.
[b]Among nonsmokers.
[c]Snuff only.

2351 cases and 8285 controls from the same data source with either cancer of the colon or rectum, cutaneous melanoma, or endocrine neoplasms had smoking histories available from medical records. Smokeless tobacco use was linked to all of the cancer subtypes studied. Adjusting for tobacco use, age, race, and sex, odds ratios associated with smokeless tobacco use were significantly elevated for cancers of the salivary glands, mouth and gum, and larynx. The large size of the series and control for other tobacco habits enhances the credibility of the findings. However, procedures for recording the tobacco data were not described, and there is the potential for serious bias if tobacco-use information was not obtained with equivalent accuracy in all case and control subgroups. The linking of smokeless tobacco with salivary gland cancer (odds ratio, 5.3; 95% confidence interval, 1.2–23.4) had not been reported previously.

The National Cancer Institute also conducted a large population-based case-control study (13). A total of 1114 oral and pharynx cancer cases from the Atlanta metropolitan area, the state of New Jersey, two counties near San Francisco, and Los Angeles County were included. Controls (n = 1268) from the same regions were selected from random-digit telephone dialing techniques or from Medicare rosters to match the age and sex distribution of cases. Among men, nearly equal percentages of cases and controls had used smokeless tobacco (6% vs. 7%, respectively). Three percent of female cases and 1% of female controls were users. Among men, distinguishing the influence of smokeless tobacco from smoked tobacco was difficult because most smokeless tobacco users smoked. Among women who did not smoke, however, a strong relationship between oral cancer and smokeless tobacco use (mostly snuff) was observed (odds ratio, 6.2; 95% confidence interval, 1.9–19.8) based on six cases and four controls.

Despite methodologic limitations, all three studies are consistent with previous epidemiologic research showing a strong relationship between upper aerodigestive tract cancers and smokeless tobacco use. Smoked tobacco could be ruled out as an explanation for the findings in the Florida report; the National Cancer Institute study as well could rule out smoking by examining the small subset of women using smokeless, but not smoked, tobacco products.

Further epidemiologic studies of smokeless tobacco and oral cancer will be difficult to mount. Case-control studies are usually the only practical study design. The major problem in conducting case-control studies is the relatively low prevalence of smokeless tobacco use among older populations who are now entering age ranges of highest cancer risk. Currently, only 3.6% of the 6.1% of American men using smokeless tobacco use it to the exclusion of other forms of tobacco, and only 0.6% of women use smokeless tobacco (14). The numbers seem likely to become even smaller, since the percentage of men aged 50 years and older who use chewing tobacco declined from 6.5% to 3.6%, and the number who use snuff declined from 2.7% to 1.6% from 1970 to 1987 (15).

There has been concern that oral cancer among young men may be on the rise in the United States. Data on men younger than 40 years of age from M. D. Anderson Cancer Center (Houston, TX) (16) and from Memorial Sloan-Kettering Cancer Center (New York, NY) (17) show an increase in the numbers of patients with tongue cancers, in the proportion of tongue cancers to all cancers, and in the percentage of patients with tongue cancer who are 40 years of age or younger. Mortality data from the United States (18) and incidence data from 10 population-based cancer registries participating in the Surveillance, Epidemiology and End Results program (19) both indicate increases in tongue cancer among younger men. However, because of limited data on tobacco habits, the role of smokeless tobacco in contributing to this rise cannot be determined.

Oral leukoplakia, a white patch that cannot be scraped off, predisposes to oral cancer. Recent studies have shown a high prevalence of such lesions in smokeless tobacco users compared with nonusers. For example, among U.S. professional baseball players attending spring training in 1988, 46% of smokeless tobacco users (averaging 5 years of use) were found to have leukoplakia compared with only 1.4% of nonusers (20). Other surveys conducted in the past few years, such as one finding a 37% prevalence of oral lesions in American Indian students in the 7th to 12th grades who used smokeless tobacco (21), confirm earlier findings of high prevalences of other lesions less severe than leukoplakia in smokeless tobacco users.

Smokeless tobacco is used in many parts of Asia in combination with other products, including lime or a combination of lime plus piper betel leaf and areca nut; the combination is called "pan" in India and is also referred to as "betel quid." In Bombay, India, oral cancer accounts for one third of all cancers, and in other areas of the world where the habit occurs, high oral cancer rates have been observed (22). The International Agency for Research on Cancer (6) concluded that there was sufficient evidence that the habit of chewing betel quid containing tobacco is carcinogenic to humans. That report cited data showing that oral leukoplakia is associated with betel quid use, that case-series reports have linked betel quid containing tobacco to oral cancer, and that a few well-conducted case-control studies with appropriate control for other risk factors showed strong dose-dependent relationships between betel quid use and oral cancer. It has not been possible to determine with certainty whether betel quid without added tobacco confers a carcinogenic risk, as this practice is less common.

Recent epidemiologic research on populations in India has continued to enhance knowledge about cancer risks associated with the use of smokeless tobacco products. One study (23) found that pan chewing increased risk of buccal and labial cancer by 13 times among males who had used chewing tobacco for 31–40 years and almost 40 times among males who had used it for 41 years or more. Corresponding relative risks among women were even higher. Studies in India have been especially useful for examining interactions among tobacco quid use and other oral cancer risk factors. Comparable studies in U.S. populations have not been able to address interactions in depth because the cancer and the "exposure" (smokeless tobacco use) are both less common. One Indian report from the 1970s suggested that smoking and unsmoked tobacco use act synergistically, raising the risk of using oral cancer from both products to a level greater than that expected based on the risks for smoking or smokeless tobacco habits alone (24). Similar findings were not supported in a recent report that compared 414 cases of oral mucosal cancer patients with 895 controls in Kerala, India. However, the investigators did find that risks were higher in persons who had begun using smokeless tobacco at younger ages than in those who had begun at older ages, suggesting some special susceptibility at younger ages. A report from India, published in 1988, concerning aerodigestive cancer showed no synergism between tobacco chewing and smoking or between chewing and alcohol consumption (25). Investigation of the joint influences of risk factors remains an important research area, in view of the strong synergism observed in epidemiologic studies of smoking and alcohol.

SMOKELESS TOBACCO–INDUCED CARCINOGENESIS

Recent research on carcinogenesis includes studies aimed at further understanding of the mechanisms of smokeless tobacco–induced carcinogenesis and on measuring and evaluating carcinogenic exposures resulting from use of smokeless tobacco, including a new focus on biologic markers of smokeless tobacco exposure.

Our understanding of the mechanisms of carcinogenesis has increased through new emphasis on the potential role of cofactors and through continued investigations of tobacco-specific nitrosamines. A potential role of cofactors has emerged through bioassays. Numerous experimental studies conducted in past decades had failed to detect oral cancers occurring in laboratory animals who had had snuff or chewing tobacco inserted in the oral cavity (2). However, in the 1980s, whole snuff applied to the lip canal in rats did result in oral tumors (26,27). More recent work in animals has shown that snuff and herpes virus may act as cocarcinogens (28) through the inhibition by snuff of type 1 herpes simplex virus DNA replication (29).

Valuable work on the mechanisms of carcinogenesis also includes research on NNK and on immunologic parameters. One recent study showed that NNK, administered subcutaneously to pregnant hamsters, led to tumors in 70% of the offspring within 1 year (30). Investigators from the American Health Foundation in New York noted that NNK is a lung carcinogen in rats, prompting them to suggest that epidemiologic studies examine the role of smokeless tobacco in the etiology of lung cancers (31). Other recent carcinogenesis studies have focused on the immune system. For example, lymphokine-activated killer activity was found to be suppressed in vitro by smokeless tobacco (32).

Estimating the dose of N-nitrosamines experienced by the smokeless tobacco user has been an active area of research since the mid-1980s. Hecht and Hoffmann have noted that the actual exposure to carcinogens experienced by the smokeless tobacco user may be a consequence of many factors (31). Considerable attention has been given to elucidating these factors. For instance, the way tobacco is processed is known to influence nitrosamine levels (31). Recently, factors such as storage conditions have been shown to profoundly influence tobacco-specific nitrosamine and other smokeless tobacco constituent levels (33). Nitrosation may take place in the saliva of smokeless tobacco users (37). A new report now shows that one of the major N-nitrosamines, NNN, is also formed from the tobacco alkaloid nornicotine under simulated in vitro stomach acid conditions (34). These studies suggest that tobacco brands, the way the product is used by the consumer, as well as individual metabolic factors may influence cancer risk.

One of the most exciting developments with respect to the internal effective dose of carcinogens received by the smokeless tobacco user has been the measurement of hemoglobin adducts of tobacco-specific N-nitrosamines. By the mid-1980s, reports had outlined the pathway, at the molecular level, by which N-nitrosamines may lead to cancer. Methylation of DNA in rat tissue has been demonstrated to result in 7-methylguanine and O^6-methylguanine, providing evidence of the defect to DNA potentially responsible for the development of cancer (35,36). However, from a practical point of view, examining DNA from tissues of smokeless tobacco users at risk for oral cancer is not feasible, and more practical approaches have to be used. This type of problem (i.e., the need for a useful surrogate measure of exposure or damage) has emerged in other health settings as well, resulting in increased emphasis on biomarkers in epidemiologic studies.

Biomarkers are "cellular, biochemical, or molecular alterations that are measurable in biological media, such as human tissues, cells, or fluids" and "may be internal indicators of exposure to external xenobiotics; they may reflect early, subclinical adverse health effects or they may define the innate susceptibility of the human host" (37). More attention is being focused on biomarkers because of their potential benefit in more precisely determining the internal dose of a carcinogen or other disease-producing agent, in assessing disease risk, and in monitoring prevention activities.

Assessments of adducts related to NNK and NNN hold considerable promise for a fuller understanding of the carcinogenic properties of smokeless tobacco because these adducts are specific to tobacco (although the sources of the tobacco exposure may be environmental smoke, smoking, or smokeless tobacco use). Examination of protein adducts in red blood cells are advantageous because they can be measured on a relatively easily obtained biologic specimen and because red blood cells have a relatively long half-life allowing estimates of usual dose. Protein-adduct levels to NNK tend to compare reasonably well with DNA-adduct levels in the less accessible target tissues for the carcinogens (38) in rats (although the relationship is complex), and the mechanism by which adducts are formed parallels that for the putative carcinogenic event itself. However, the exact relationship between adduct levels and the actual carcinogenic events themselves is not clear, and the correspondence between adduct levels and actual disease risk in humans remains to be evaluated.

In work to date, levels of hemoglobin adducts to tobacco-specific N-nitrosamine compounds were found to be more than 15 times higher in smokeless tobacco users than in nonusers of tobacco, and more than six times higher in smokeless tobacco users than in smokers (39). Discovering more about the human behavioral factors influencing adduct levels will be valuable. DNA adduct levels in other materials (e.g., oral mucosal cells) have also been examined in a population of tobacco chewers in India, but no differences in adduct levels were found when users were compared with nonusers (40).

Hemoglobin adducts are not the only biomarker that has been used to monitor damage from smokeless tobacco in the target tissues at risk for oral cancer. The mean number of micronuclei, counted in exfoliated buccal mucosal cells, also have been found to be higher in groups of tobacco chewers than in groups of nonusers. Micronuclei are also influenced by substances thought to modulate cancer risk such as β-carotene (41). Micronuclei are a generalized marker of damage and are not specific to tobacco products. The link with disease outcomes has not been measured, and the mechanism by which micronuclei are formed is not specifically related to the carcinogenic process. However, exfoliated cells from the buccal mucosa are readily obtained through noninvasive means.

CONCLUSIONS

Three recent epidemiologic studies continue to show that smokeless tobacco confers upon its users an increased risk of oral cavity cancers. For the first time, one of these studies linked smokeless tobacco use to cancers of the salivary glands, and it also showed links between smokeless tobacco use and other upper aerodigestive tract cancers. Laboratory work has further refined our understanding of the carcinogenic process by identifying potential cocarcinogens and new routes of exposure (e.g., transplacental carcinogenesis). Hemoglobin adduct measurements may prove to be extremely useful markers of the dose of carcinogens experienced by the smokeless tobacco user.

Although difficult to conduct, epidemiologic studies are needed of other cancer sites where associations with smokeless tobacco use have been noted (e.g., pancreas, nasal), but where conclusive findings have been elusive. In view of reports on lung cancers in animals exposed to NNK, epidemiologic studies of lung cancer should include questionnaire material on smokeless tobacco.

Adapting hemoglobin adduct assays to larger-scale epidemiologic surveys and including other biologic markers in such surveys will help to elucidate behavioral and metabolic factors influencing adduct levels; this may help in identifying individuals at highest risk for cancer. More research on the long-term implications of high adduct levels in laboratory animals will be important in making extrapolations to cancer risks in human populations.

REFERENCES

1. Schuman LM. Patterns of smoking behavior. NIDA Monograph 17:36–66, 1977.
2. Advisory Committee to the Surgeon General. The Health Consequences of Using Smokeless Tobacco (NIH Publication No. 86-2874). Bethesda, MD: U.S. Department of Health and Human Services, 1986, p. 7.
3. U.S. Department of Agriculture. Tobacco Situation. No. TS215. June 1991.
4. Winn DM, Blot WJ, Shy CM, Pickle LW, Toledo A, Fraumeni JF Jr. Snuff dipping and oral cancer among women in the southern United States. N Engl J Med 304:745–749, 1981.
5. Mason TJ, McKay FW, Hoover R, Blot WJ, Fraumeni JF Jr. Atlas of cancer mortality for U.S. counties, 1950–69 (NIH Publication No. 75-780). Bethesda, MD: U.S. Department of Health and Human Services, 1975, p. 37.
6. International Agency for Research on Cancer. IARC Monographs on the Evaluation of the Carcinogenic Risk of Chemicals to Humans: Tobacco Habits Other Than Smoking; Betel-quid and Areca-nut Chewing; and Some Related Nitrosamines. Vol. 37. Lyon, France: International Agency for Research on Cancer, 1985, pp. 37–136.
7. Hoffmann D, Hecht SS. Nicotine-derived N-nitrosamines and tobacco-related cancer: Current status and future directions. Cancer Res 45:935–944, 1985.

8. Hoffmann D, Adams JD, Lisk D, Fisenne I, Brunnemann KD. Toxic and carcinogenic agents in dry and moist snuff. J Natl Cancer Inst 79:1281–1286, 1987.
9. National Institutes of Health Consensus Development Conference Statement. Health Implications of Smokeless Tobacco. Vol. 6, No. 1. Bethesda, MD: National Institutes of Health, 1986.
10. Comprehensive Smokeless Tobacco Health Education Act of 1986. Public Law 99-252. February 27, 1986.
11. Spitz MR, Fueger JJ, Goepfert H, Hong WK, Newell GR. Squamous cell carcinoma of the upper aerodigestive tract: A case comparison analysis. Cancer 61:203–208, 1988.
12. Stockwell HG, Lyman GH. Impact of smoking and smokeless tobacco on the risk of cancer of the head and neck. Head Neck Surg 9:104–110, 1986.
13. Blot WJ, McLaughlin JK, Winn DM, Austin DF, Greenberg RS, Preston-Martin S, Bernstein L. Schoenberg JB, Stemhagen A, Fraumeni JF Jr. Smoking and drinking in relation to oral and pharyngeal cancer. Cancer Res 48:3282–3287, 1988.
14. Schoenborn CA, Boyd G. Smoking and other tobacco use: United States, 1987. National Center for Health Statistics. Vital Health Stat 10(169), 1989.
15. U.S. Department of Health and Human Services. Reducing the Health Consequences of Smoking: 25 Years of Progress. A Report of the Surgeon General (DHHS Publication No. (CDC) 89-8411). Rockville, MD: U.S. Department of Health and Human Services, 1989, p. 320.
16. Schantz SP, Byers RM, Goepfert H. Tobacco and cancer of the tongue in young adults (letter). JAMA 259:1943–1944, 1988.
17. Shemen LJ, Klotz J, Schottenfeld D, Strong EW. Increase of tongue cancer in young men (letter). JAMA 252:1857, 1984.
18. Depue RH. Rising mortality from cancer of the tongue in young white males (letter). N Engl J Med 315:647, 1986.
19. Davis S, Severson RK. Increasing incidence of cancer of the tongue in the United States among young adults (letter). Lancet 2:910–911, 1987.
20. Ernster VL, Grady DG, Greene JC, Walsh M, Robertson P, Daniels TE, Benowitz N, Siegel D, Gerbert B, Hauck WW. Smokeless tobacco use and health effects among baseball players. JAMA 264:218–224, 1990.
21. Prevalence of oral lesions and smokeless tobacco use in Northern Plains Indians. MMWR 37:608–611, 1988.
22. Desai PB. Problems and challenges due to tobacco-related cancer: A clinical perspective. Presented at the International Symposium on the Control of Tobacco-Related Cancers and Other Diseases. Bombay, India January 15–19, 1990.
23. Sankaranarayanan R, Duffy SW, Padmakumary G, Day NE, Nari MK. Risk factors for cancer of the buccal and labial mucosa in Kerala, Southern India. J Epidemiol Community Health 44:286–292, 1990.
24. Jayant K, Balakrishnan V, Sanghvi LD, Jussawalla DJ. Quantification of the role of smoking and chewing tobacco in oral, pharyngeal and oesophageal cancers. Br J Cancer 35:232–235, 1977.
25. Notani PN. Role of alcohol in cancer of the upper alimentary tract: Use of models in risk assessment. J Epidemiol Community Health 42:187–192, 1988.
26. Hirsch JM, Hohansson SL. Effect of long-term application of snuff on oral mucosa: An experimental study in the rat. J Oral Pathol 12:187–198, 1983.
27. Hecht SS, Rivenson A, Braley J, DiBello J, Adams JD, Hoffmann D. Induction of oral cavity tumors in F344 rats by tobacco-specific nitrosamines and snuff. Cancer Res 46:4162–4166, 1986.
28. Park N-H, Sapp JP, Herbosa EG. Oral cancer induced in hamsters with herpes simplex infection and simulated snuff dipping. Oral Surg Oral Med Oral Pathol 62:164–168, 1986.
29. Oh JS, Cherrick HM, Park N-H. Effect of snuff extract on the replication and synthesis of viral DNA and proteins in cells infected with herpes simplex virus. J Oral Maxillofac Surg 48:373–379, 1990.
30. Correa E, Joshi PV, Castonguay A, Schuller HM. The tobacco-specific nitrosamine 4-(methylnitrosamino)-1-(3-pyridyl)-1-butanone is an active transplacental carcinogen in Syrian golden hamsters. Cancer Res 50:3435–3438, 1990.
31. Hecht SS, Hoffmann D. Tobacco-specific nitrosamines: An important group of carcinogens in tobacco and tobacco smoke. Carcinogenesis 9:875–884, 1988.
32. Lindemann RA, Park NH. Inhibition of human lymphokine-activated killer activity by smokeless tobacco (snuff) extract. Arch Oral Biol 33:317–321, 1988.
33. Anderson RA, Burton HR, Fleming PD, Hamilton-Kemp TR. Effect of storage conditions on nitrosated, acylated, and oxidized pyridine alkaloid derivatives in smokeless tobacco products. Cancer Res 49:5895-5900, 1989.
34. Tricker AR, Haubner R, Spiegelhalder B, Preussmann R. The occurrence of tobacco-specific nitrosamines in oral tobacco products and their potential formation under simulated gastric conditions. Food Chem Toxicol 26:861–865, 1988.
35. Hecht SS, Trushin N, Castonguay A, Rivenson A. Comparative carcinogenicity and DNA methylation in F344 rats by 4-(methylnitrosamino)-1-(3-pyridyl)-1-butanone and N-nitrosodimethylamine. Cancer Res 46:498–502, 1986.

36. Castonguay A, Tharp R, Hecht SS. Kinetics of DNA methylation by the tobacco-specific carcinogen 4-(methylnitrosamino)-1-(3-pyridyl)-1-butanone in the F344 rat. In O'Neill IK, von Borstel RC, Miller CT, Long JT, Bartsch H (eds): *N-Nitroso Compounds: Occurrence, Biological Effects and Relevance to Human Cancer.* IARC Scientific Publications No. 57. Lyon, France: International Agency for Research on Cancer, 1984, pp. 787–796.

37. Hulka BS. Overview of biological markers. In Hulka BS, Wilcosky TC, Griffith JD (eds): *Biological Markers in Epidemiology.* New York: Oxford University Press, 1990, pp. 3–4.

38. Murphy SE, Palomino A, Hecht SS, Hoffmann D. A dose response study of DNA adduct formation and hemoglobin adduct formation of 4-(methylnitrosamino)-1-(3-pyridyl)-1-butanone in F344 rats. Cancer Res 50:5446–5452, 1990.

39. Carmella SG, Kagan SS, Kagan M, Foiles PG, Palladino G, Quart AM, Quart E, Hecht SS. Mass spectrometric analysis of tobacco-specific nitrosamine hemoglobin adducts in snuff dippers, smokers, and nonsmokers. Cancer Res 50:5438–5445, 1990.

40. Chack M, Gupta RC. Evaluation of DNA damage in the oral mucosa of tobacco users and non-users by ^{32}P-adduct assay. Carcinogenesis 9:2309–2313, 1988.

41. Stich HF, Dunn BP. DNA adducts, micronuclei, and leukoplakias as intermediate endpoints in intervention trials. In Bartsch H, Hemminki K, O'Neill IK. *Methods for Detecting DNA Damaging Agents in Humans: Applications in Cancer Epidemiology and Prevention.* IARC Scientific Publications No. 89. Lyon, France: International Agency for Research on Cancer, 1988, pp. 137–145.

Biologic Markers as Predictors of Risk in Aerodigestive Tract Cancers

Bruce Trock

Division of Population Science
Fox Chase Cancer Center
Cheltenham, Pennsylvania

The goal of research on biologic markers is to develop methods to reliably distinguish individuals at high risk for an adverse outcome. Ideally, the ability to so classify individuals should improve the probability of intervening to avoid or reduce the severity of the outcome. For aerodigestive tract cancers, the following applications for biologic markers may be considered, each with different implications for intervention: (a) Early detection of disease in asymptomatic individuals with such markers would allow treatment with the highest probability of cure and fewest adverse effects. (b) Predicting the probability of recurrence or second primary tumor prior to therapy by using biologic markers that could identify relapse-prone individuals, particularly if they could discriminate subgroups within categories of established prognostic factors, would permit more effective targeting of aggressive therapy and intensive surveillance. (c) Monitoring response to therapy with markers that exhibit dynamic changes with disease progression may permit detection of relapse in early, possibly preclinical, stages.

A large number of potential markers for aerodigestive tract cancers have been identified. However, none has been widely tested to date, and most have been studied in small samples. Nevertheless, many of these markers appear very promising. The discussion that follows will describe the evidence for a number of these markers. In addition to describing the associations between levels of a particular marker and tumor behavior, the discussion will also highlight the degree to which interpretation of results is limited by aspects of the study design.

This is not meant to be an exhaustive review of all biologic markers of aerodigestive tract cancers. The focus will be on markers that, at this early stage of testing, appear to have strong potential for use in individual patients to predict prognosis or monitor response to treatment. Biomarkers for screening or early detection will not be discussed because the health practices of a large proportion of those at high risk for aerodigestive tract cancers limit the feasibility of screening for preclinical disease with current approaches. However, some of the markers that will be described with respect to predicting prognosis or monitoring response to therapy also do well at discriminating between patients with aerodigestive tract cancers and normal controls.

Before describing individual biomarkers, three important general criteria for biomarker validity and usefulness in head and neck cancer should be briefly reviewed: (a) The marker must accurately discriminate between individuals at high risk (or in early stages) of adverse disease outcome. Thus, the marker will be able to identify a high proportion of individuals who will undergo or who are in early stages of relapse (high sensitivity), and identify a high

The Biology and Prevention of Aerodigestive Tract Cancers
Edited by G.R.Newell and W.K. Hong, Plenum Press, New York, 1992

47

proportion who will not undergo relapse or who have stable disease (high specificity). (b) The biomarker must exhibit a quantitative association with stage of disease, prognosis, or tumor burden. Thus, increases (or decreases) in the marker will be associated with more advanced or aggressive disease, or disease progression. (c) The biomarker must be measured in small samples and should be relatively quick, inexpensive, and noninvasive (1,2).

Of the three criteria, the first is generally the most difficult to satisfy. To be clinically useful, biomarkers must allow prediction of outcome in individual patients with high accuracy. However, a common criticism of biomarker research is that many biologic markers have relatively low sensitivity, low specificity, or both. Thus, for markers that are positively correlated with risk, many individuals with aggressive or progressive disease will have low marker levels, while many with low risk or stable disease will have elevated levels.

Unfortunately, there is a trade-off between the sensitivity and specificity of biomarkers; increases in one parameter are made at the expense of decreases in the other. Most biomarkers are measured on a continuum, with a more or less arbitrary cut point determining the level at which individuals are considered to have abnormal or high-risk values. Choosing a less stringent cut point increases sensitivity but also increases false positives or decreases specificity. More stringent cut points have the opposite effect. Both sensitivity and specificity can be increased by using a panel of biomarkers, but a trade-off is still required. Sensitivity is increased by judging a test result to be abnormal if any of several biomarkers exhibits an abnormal value. Conversely, specificity is increased by requiring multiple markers to exhibit abnormal values before the test result is judged abnormal.

However, a decision regarding the trade-off between these two test criteria can be made by considering some of the characteristics of aerodigestive tract cancer and the types of biomarker applications described above (i.e., predicting prognosis and monitoring response to therapy). When using a biomarker or other test to discriminate among two mutually exclusive groups, the probability of misclassification (P(M) = rate of false positives + false negatives) is a function of sensitivity (SE), specificity (SP), and the prevalence (PR) of the adverse outcome, as follows (3):

$$P(M) = PR (1 - SE) + (1 - PR) (1 - SP).$$

Typically, we think of using a biomarker to screen for early detection of a disease of low prevalence. However, for patients with aerodigestive tract cancer, the rate of relapse or second primaries is fairly high. The effect of these differences in prevalence on misclassification can be illustrated with a hypothetical example of a biomarker of high sensitivity (SE = 0.85) and low specificity (SP = 0.50). The equation above reveals that when prevalence is low (e.g., PR = 0.10), the probability of misclassification is 0.47. However, for a higher prevalence, such as that observed for relapse of aerodigestive tract cancer (PR = 0.60), the misclassification rate drops to 0.29. Thus, for biomarkers of aerodigestive tract cancer, it may be feasible to relax the constraint for specificity to achieve greater sensitivity without risking a high rate of misclassification. This is particularly true if markers are used to target individuals for more intensive surveillance or to monitor response to therapy; the "cost" associated with a false-positive classification is relatively minor.

In the discussion that follows, the ability of the biomarkers to satisfy criteria (a) and (b) above will be emphasized (all of the biomarkers satisfy criterion [c]).

BIOMARKERS FOR PREDICTING PROGNOSIS

For these markers, crude estimates of sensitivity and specificity that were calculated by this author are presented, based on data in the published reports. These estimates are clearly dependent on the length of follow-up in any given study and may change with longer follow-up. However, in these studies, follow-up was long enough to reveal significant differences in risk of relapse, suggesting that these markers are at least sufficient for predicting more aggressive tumor behavior.

In Vitro Bleomycin Sensitivity

This cytogenetic assay quantifies chromosome breakage in lymphocyte cultures in response to bleomycin treatment. It is hypothesized that sensitivity to the genotoxic effects of bleomycin is indicative of DNA-repair capability and overall susceptibility to mutagenic agents. Individuals are classified according to the average number of chromosome breaks per cell as nonsensitive (<0.80 breaks), sensitive (≥0.80 breaks), or hypersensitive (>1.0 breaks). Approximately 23% and 12% of healthy individuals are sensitive and hypersensitive, respectively (4).

In a comparison of patients with aerodigestive tract cancer and a convenience sample of controls (hospital employees and patients' spouses), chromosome sensitivity was associated with excess risk: odds ratio (OR) = 3.9 (1.6, 9.1) after adjusting for age, sex, smoking status and alcohol use. Chromosome sensitivity was a risk factor even in the absence of smoking or drinking. Although the controls were not a representative random sample of the healthy population, the distribution of chromosome sensitivity was similar to that seen in a more representative control sample. Furthermore, adjustment for other characteristics associated with aerodigestive tract cancer risk minimized the potential for confounding (4).

The bleomycin assay was also used to assess the risk of second primary tumors among a group of previously untreated patients with aerodigestive tract cancer. It was hypothesized that deficient DNA-repair capability would result in increased risk of second or multiple primaries among these patients, based on the concept of field cancerization. After an average of 20 months of follow-up (range, 4–31 months), patients exhibiting bleomycin hypersensitivity (>1.0 breaks per cell) had a relative risk (RR) of 3.5 for developing multiple primary tumors ($P < 0.05$). The two groups (hypersensitive and not hypersensitive) exhibited no statistically significant differences in length of follow-up, age, sex, treatment, or use of tobacco or alcohol (5). Based on the number of patients with second primary tumors in each group, this author calculated a sensitivity of 0.69 and a specificity of 0.66 for testing the risk of multiple primary tumors. The study did not discuss whether the rate of recurrence differed between the two groups.

A9 Cell Membrane Antigen

Because the A9 antigen is found in the germinal layer of normal epithelial cells but not in mature keratinocytes, it is associated with the replicating cell compartment. It appears to be expressed in all squamous cell cancers and is a member of the integrin superfamily of extracellular receptors, which are associated with invasiveness and metastatic potential. Three distinct immunohistochemical staining patterns are discernible, representing increasing antigen expression. The antigen is expressed at higher levels in tumor cells than in normal epithelium and is higher in cell lines derived from metastatic tumor than those from primary tumor in the same patient. Thus, the staining pattern of this antigen correlates with tumor aggressiveness (6).

In a sample of 82 consecutive, previously untreated patients with aerodigestive tract cancer, antigen expression was assessed at the interface between normal and tumor tissue, at the time of primary surgery. Risk of recurrence was significantly increased among patients expressing high levels of A9 antigen at diagnosis: RR = 1.7 (calculated by this author). This increase in risk was independent of tumor size, stage, or nodal status at diagnosis. The length of the disease-free survival interval was also shorter for individuals with high A9 expression. Among those with the highest staining pattern, the median disease-free interval was 10 months; median survival had not been reached after more than 20 months of follow-up in the patients exhibiting the two lower staining patterns ($P < 0.05$) (6). As a marker of recurrence potential, A9 expression exhibited a sensitivity of 0.72 and a specificity of 0.51. Surprisingly, A9 expression was correlated with low tumor grade and increased differentiation, which are typically associated with less aggressive tumors. This may be because of lower DNA content in metastatic tumors than in primary tumors from the same individuals; nuclear grade could be lower due to smaller, less hyperchromatic nuclei (6). However, this also points to the ability of the A9 antigen to discern a high-risk subset of tumors among patients with other characteristics that appear favorable.

Blood-Group Antigens (A, B, H)

In addition to the role of A9 antigen, expression of the A, B, and H blood-group antigens was also examined in the same group of patients. In contrast with the A9 antigen, the blood-group antigens are expressed in the suprabasal keratinocytes in normal tissue; thus, they are associated with the differentiated state. Compared with normal squamous epithelium, squamous cell carcinomas exhibit loss of expression of these blood-group antigens. Among patients with aerodigestive tract cancer, significant associations were observed between loss of expression and low tumor grade, but not with tumor stage, growth pattern, degree of differentiation, or A9-antigen expression. As with A9 antigen, blood-group expression was assessed at the tumor-normal tissue interface (6).

Patients exhibiting loss of blood-group antigen expression had a significantly increased risk of recurrence (RR = 2.1). These patients also had decreased disease-free survival time; median disease-free interval was 7 months in the group with loss of expression, while median survival in the group expressing blood-group antigens had not been reached after 50 months (6). As a recurrence marker, loss of blood-group expression exhibited a sensitivity of 0.53, with a specificity of 0.84 (calculated by this author).

These investigators also examined the joint expression of blood-group and A9 antigens. Risk of recurrence for individuals with high A9 expression and loss of blood-group antigens was significantly increased (RR = 3.2). Disease-free survival was significantly decreased in individuals with either high A9 expression, loss of blood-group antigen, or both, compared with individuals with low A9 expression and retention of blood-group antigen ($P = 0.007$). In a proportional hazards model that examined the independent effect of these markers, after adjusting for tumor site, stage, and lymph node involvement, the most powerful predictor of survival was the combination of low A9 expression and retention of blood-group antigen ($P = 0.01$). The recurrence rate in this group (24%) was less than half that of individuals without this favorable combination (58%) (6). By combining these two markers, sensitivity was increased to 0.85, while specificity dropped to 0.49. Thus, these two markers may be excellent candidates for use in a panel approach.

c-*myc* Oncogene Expression

In a small series of squamous cell tumors of the head and neck, expression of the c-*myc* oncogene was found to be elevated in tumor tissue when compared with that found in the normal tissue margin. Furthermore, expression of this oncogene exhibited a statistically significant increase with tumor stage ($P < 0.05$). The increase in expression did not appear to be the result of gene amplification. Expression was not associated with any other clinicopathologic characteristics (7). However, six of these tumor specimens came from recurrences in patients previously treated with radiotherapy for primary tumor, so it is difficult to assess the significance of the observed results.

In a subsequent study using a larger sample, these investigators again observed higher levels of expression in tumor than in normal tissue, and an association with tumor stage, but not with nodal status, differentiation, grade, site, age, or sex. Instead of measuring c-*myc* mRNA, the investigators used an ELISA technique to quantify the amount of the *myc*-derived p62 protein, an approach with greater sensitivity and reproducibility (8).

Patients with levels of p62 protein more than two standard deviations above the mean for expression in normal tissue exhibited increased risk of recurrence or death from disease (RR = 3.7). They also had a significant decrease in survival, with median survival of 36 months, compared with approximately 80% survival at 36 months among patients with normal *myc* levels ($P < 0.02$) (8). The sensitivity of this marker for recurrence or death from disease was 0.77, with a specificity of 0.65.

There are some methodologic concerns with this study that may affect interpretation. Of the 44 patients in the study, 21 were undergoing surgery for recurrent disease at the time of c-*myc* determination. There is no information in the report about prior radiotherapy for these patients. However, the level of c-*myc* expression in patients with recurrent tumors at the start of the study did not differ significantly from that of patients with primary tumors, suggesting that radiotherapy was not likely to have influenced gene expression. A more serious concern is that the analysis was not adjusted for the effects of other prognostic factors. Because the tumor stage was higher in patients with elevated c-*myc* expression, there is no way to know if the gene has prognostic value independently of tumor stage. A stratified analysis to show the effect of c-*myc* expression separately for Stage I–II and Stage III–IV patients would resolve this issue.

Although preliminary, the results for the four biomarkers described above suggest that they may be useful for discriminating tumors with more aggressive behavior. The crude sensitivity values calculated from the published data suggest that fairly high sensitivity may be attainable with panels of these markers. This was also apparent from the gain in sensitivity observed for the combination of A9 and blood-group antigens. The fact that these markers tend not to be associated with most established prognostic factors suggests that, if the current results are representative, they may be useful for defining high-risk subgroups within previously recognized prognostic categories. Clearly, these results need to be replicated in larger samples, using multiple markers and more complete analytic techniques to control for confounding.

MARKERS OF RESPONSE TO THERAPY

This class of markers is associated with tumor burden and disease progression. Unlike the markers described above, interindividual variability in marker levels may be high for these markers, making it difficult or impossible to establish a cut point. Thus, these markers will not be discussed in terms of sensitivity and specificity. However, the correlation between changes from baseline levels and tumor burden or progression allows these to be used in a serial fashion. Serial measurements of these markers before therapy and throughout follow-up would reveal dynamic changes in levels corresponding to reduction of tumor burden following successful therapy, and increases corresponding to recurrence or second primary tumors.

Serum Ferritin

This protein is typically measured in serum using enzyme-immunoassay or related techniques. Among a group of normal controls, levels tended to increase in patients who were older, smoked, and were male (the increase due to gender was not statistically significant). In comparison with controls, patients with aerodigestive tract cancer had significantly higher serum ferritin levels. Levels in aerodigestive tract cancer patients were similar to levels observed for lung, breast, and colon cancer patients. However, interindividual variation was high, with many controls exhibiting high levels, and some patients with advanced disease exhibiting low levels. Levels among patients with disease stages III–IV were higher than among those with stages I–II (9). Similar results were seen in another study, although the association with stage was not assessed (10).

Serum ferritin levels in individual patients tended to decrease following successful therapy. This was determined by comparing pre- and posttherapeutic levels in those who had recurrences within the first year following therapy with those who remained free of disease. Individuals who suffered recurrences tended to exhibit levels that increased or remained high (relative to controls). Even among patients who were disease free at more than 12 months posttherapy (9,10) and among a group of patients disease free for more than 5 years (9), the levels were greater than those among normal controls. However, this may reflect resumption of cigarette smoking at higher levels among the patients than among the controls. Levels in controls who were followed longitudinally did not change, and there were no differences in serum iron levels between cases and controls (9).

Protein-Bound Sialic Acid

Sialic acid levels of glycoproteins and glycolipids in cell membranes and surfaces are increased in malignant cells from a number of tumor sites including aerodigestive tract, lung, breast, prostate, and bladder. Characteristics of cell surfaces and membranes affect characteristics of tumor behavior such as cell-to-cell recognition, adhesion, antigenicity, and invasiveness. Glycoproteins are shed into the blood from tumor-cell surfaces, allowing the serum to be assayed for sialic acid content.

A series of 165 patients with tumors of the head and neck were compared to 50 age-matched controls. No significant differences were seen for lipid-bound sialic acid, but protein-bound sialic acid (PBSA) levels were higher in patients than in normal controls. A trend was observed with extent of disease at diagnosis, with levels of PBSA increasing progressively as follows: normal < primary tumor < lymph node metastasis < distant metastasis ($P < 0.0001$) (11). PBSA levels were also higher in patients with poorly differentiated tumors than in those with moderately or well-differentiated tumors. No data were given on the association of PBSA with other clinical or tumor characteristics, or patient characteristics such as age, gender, or tobacco use. This clearly must be done to determine the independent value of PBSA.

Among a subgroup of 23 patients, serial measurements indicated that PBSA decreased 2–4 weeks following surgery among patients who remained disease free after the fifth posttreatment follow-up visit, and increased or remained high in those who suffered recurrent disease. However, only two patients from this subgroup remained disease free for this time period (11). Furthermore, there is no indication of how this subgroup was chosen for follow-up with serial PBSA. Thus, replication of these results in larger, more carefully controlled studies is necessary.

Serum Enzymes

Serum levels of a number of enzymes have been shown to differ in patients with aerodigestive tract cancer versus controls and to vary with extent and progression of disease. Altered serum levels may arise in a number of ways, including increased liberation of intracellular enzymes associated with rapid proliferation of tumor cells, or as a result of abnormal biochemical processes associated with the malignant phenotype (1). Changes in levels of the following enzymes have been shown to correlate (positively or negatively, as shown) with tumor burden, response to therapy, and recurrence (1,12):

(a) Dipeptidyl peptidase IV (DPP-IV) activity (negative correlation);
(b) Aliesterase (negative correlation);
(c) Phosphohexose isomerase (positive correlation);
(d) Adenosine deaminase (positive correlation).

Similar results have been observed with all of these enzymes. Only DPP-IV will be discussed here, as it was tested in the largest group of patients and because similar results were seen in patients and an animal model (12).

DPP-IV is actually an enzyme that hydrolyzes N-terminal X-proline from peptides in rat liver and kidney. But, this enzyme activity has also been demonstrated in human sera, and it exhibits quantitative changes with a number of disorders. A sample of 51 oral cancer patients exhibited significantly lower levels of DPP-IV activity than 66 age- and gender-matched healthy controls ($P < 0.001$). However, there was no association with stage of disease among patients. Levels tended to increase following therapy (surgery, radiation, or chemotherapy) and remained high for those patients who were still disease free more than 2 years following treatment. However, among patients with relapse in less than 2 years, levels tended to decrease or remain low following therapy (12). Again, there was no assessment of the influence of other prognostic factors, so more carefully controlled studies will be required for further assessment of this marker.

An animal model also supported the use of DPP-IV activity as a marker of response to therapy and progression. In both nude mice and hamsters inoculated with tumor cells, DPP-IV activity decreased as tumor weight increased. Resection of tumor led to an increase in DPP-IV, which subsequently decreased with recurrence. No change in DPP-IV activity was observed for animals that underwent a sham operation (12).

As with the biomarkers of prognosis discussed above, markers used to monitor response to therapy exhibit great potential for use in panels, with baseline and serial measurements used to detect relapse at its earliest stages. Even though the relation between other prognostic factors and markers of response to therapy was not assessed, it is likely that these markers will be useful because of their dynamic response to changes in disease status.

CONCLUSION

A number of biologic markers exhibit great potential for use in predicting prognosis, tumor behavior, and response to therapy. Because none of them exhibits really high sensitivity, they may be more appropriately used in panels, although false-positive results (low specificity) will still be a concern in using these markers to target patients for more aggressive therapy. Biomarkers will be particularly important if they can discern subgroups at high risk for relapse within categories of established prognostic factors. The potential to use markers both to identify the subgroup of patients at high risk for relapse and to monitor them for early signs of relapse is especially provocative.

The results discussed above require verification in larger, more detailed studies. Many promising biomarkers (micronuclei, squamous cell differentiation markers, and cellular proliferation markers) were not included in this review. Micronuclei may be more appropriate for screening and early detection, while differentiation and proliferation markers exhibit complex expression patterns that are not easily translatable to high sensitivity or specificity at this time (2). Other markers may also be promising, but they either have low sensitivity or have been less widely tested (13–17).

REFERENCES

1. Hanna EYN, Papay FA, Gupta MK, Lavertu P, Tucker HM. Serum tumor markers of head and neck cancer: Current status. Head Neck 12:50–59, 1990.
2. Lippman SM, Lee JS, Lotan R, Hittelman W, Wargovich MJ, Hong WK. Biomarkers as intermediate end points in chemoprevention trials. J Natl Cancer Inst 82:7;555–560, 1990.
3. Makuch RW, Muenz LR. Evaluating the adequacy of tumor markers to discriminate among distinct populations. Semin Oncol 14:89–101, 1987.

4. Spitz MR, Fueger JJ, Beddingfield NA, Annegers JF, Hsu TC, Newell GR, Schantz SP. Chromosome sensitivity to bleomycin-induced mutagenesis, an independent risk factor for upper aerodigestive tract cancers. Cancer Res 49:4626–4628, 1989.

5. Schantz SP, Spitz MR, Hsu TC. Mutagen sensitivity in patients with head and neck cancers: A biologic marker for risk of multiple primary malignancies. J Natl Cancer Inst 82:1773–1775, 1990.

6. Wolf GT, Carey TE, Schmaltz SP, McClatchey KD, Poore J, Glaser L, Hayashida DJS, Hsu S. Altered antigen expression predicts outcome in squamous cell carcinoma of the head and neck. J Natl Cancer Inst 82:1566–1572, 1990.

7. Field JK, Lamothe A, Spandidos DA. Clinical relevance of oncogene expression in head and neck tumors. Anticancer Res 6:595–600, 1986.

8. Field JK, Spandidos DA, Stell PM, Vaughan ED, Evan GI, Moore JP. Elevated expression of the c-*myc* oncoprotein correlates with poor prognosis in head and neck squamous cell carcinoma. Oncogene 4:1463–1468, 1989.

9. Maxim PE, Veltri RW. Serum ferritin as a tumor marker in patients with squamous cell carcinoma of the head and neck. Cancer 57:305–311, 1986.

10. Bhatavdekar JM, Vora HH, Goyal A, Shah NG, Karelia NH, Trivedi SN. Significance of ferritin as a marker in head and neck malignancies. Tumori 73:59–63, 1987.

11. Bhatavdekar JM, Vora HH, Patel DD. Serum sialic acid forms as markers for head and neck malignancies. Neoplasma 35:425–434, 1988.

12. Urade M, Komatsu M, Yamaoka M, Fukasawa K, Harada M, Mima T, Matsuya T. Serum dipeptidyl peptidase activities as a possible marker of oral cancer. Cancer 64:1274–1280, 1989.

13. Berenson JR, Yang J, Mickel RA. Frequent amplification of the *bcl*-1 locus in head and neck squamous cell carcinomas. Oncogene 4:1111–1116, 1989.

14. Caldani C, Thyss A, Schneider M, Milano G, Buray L, Demard F. Orosomucoid: Prealbumin ratio—A marker of the host-tumor relationship in head and neck cancer. Eur J Cancer Clin Oncol 24:653–657, 1988.

15. Remani P, Ankathil R, Vijayan KK, Beevi H, Rajendran R, Vijayakumar T. Circulating immune complexes as an immunological marker in premalignant and malignant lesions of the oral cavity. Cancer Lett 40:185–191, 1988.

16. Rubin AL, Parenteau NL, Rice RH. Coordination of keratinocyte programming in human SCC-13 squamous carcinoma and normal epidermal cells. J Cell Physiol 138:208–214, 1989.

17. Schantz SP, Savage HE, Brown BW, Young G, Liu FJ, Reger G, Newman RA. Significance of C1q-binding macromolecules within the head and neck cancer patient. Cancer Res 50:4349–4354, 1990.

Hamster Lung Cancer Model of Carcinogenesis and Chemoprevention

Richard C. Moon,[1] Kandala V.N. Rao,[1] Carol J. Detrisac,[1] and Gary J. Kelloff[2]

[1]*Life Sciences Research*
IIT Research Institute
Chicago, Illinois

[2]*Chemoprevention Branch*
National Cancer Institute
Bethesda, Maryland

INTRODUCTION

Attempts to establish a lung cancer model in hamsters that is histologically and biochemically similar to bronchogenic carcinoma in man have had limited success (1,2) Earlier hamster and mouse studies employed methods such as thread transfixions (3,4) and exposure to radioactive compounds either by inhalation (5) or implantation of intrabronchia. pellets (6). Lung cancer models in hamsters employed by Saffiotti and his associates (7–10) required the intratracheal instillation of suspensions of a crystalline polycyclic aromatic hydrocarbon adsorbed to carrier particles of inert dust. The use of nitroso-compounds, with and without carrier dust, to induce tracheal and pulmonary lesions in hamsters has also been employed (11–15). However, the physiochemical properties of these carcinogens, such as solubility and particle size, and the nature of the carrier particles are very critical with regard to tumor induction. As a result, the feasibility of obtaining a reproducible incidence of respiratory cancer in different laboratories using these techniques appears remote. Furthermore, many of the earlier lung tumor models exhibited a very low cancer incidence and a long latency period.

In our laboratory, we have used two tumor models for lung cancer that permit the rapid evaluation of potential chemopreventive agents. The requirements were that the models induce a reproducibly low and high incidence of respiratory cancers within a short period (5 months), that they produce neoplastic lesions in a relatively localized area so that histologic processing would be minimal, that they be simple enough that large numbers of animals could be treated, and that they have little if any toxic effects.

Tracheobronchial Cancer Model (*N*-methyl-*N*-nitrosourea/Syrian Golden Hamster)

The induction of invasive cancers in a localized area of the hamster trachea by the carcinogen *N*-methyl-*N*-nitrosourea (MNU) was originally described by Schreiber et al. (16),

The Biology and Prevention of Aerodigestive Tract Cancers
Edited by G.R.Newell and W.K. Hong, Plenum Press, New York, 1992

55

but we have substantially modified both the equipment and the methodology for use in chemoprevention studies (17). This model for respiratory cancer eliminates many of the problems inherent in the benzo[a]pyrene/ferric oxide model for lung tumor induction in hamsters.

Through the use of a specially designed catheter, the area of tissue exposed to MNU is limited to a defined region of the trachea; tumors develop only in the exposed area of the trachea. Because organ exposure is limited to a known area, quantitation of doses is facilitated. MNU is delivered and reabsorbed by the catheter using no carrier particles; thus, any possible influence of particle size, composition, or method of carcinogen/carrier preparation is eliminated. Studies completed in this laboratory have developed dosing regimens that yield a reproducible tumor response with little or no toxic effect. Serial kill studies have characterized the histogenesis of the carcinogen-induced lesions (18) and provided a relevant time frame for the development of MNU-induced tracheal cancer. The lesions show a characteristic histogenic pattern of goblet cell hyperplasia and loss of ciliated cells, followed by squamous metaplasia with increasing stratification, carcinoma in situ, and invasive carcinoma (19).

The staff at IIT Research Institute redesigned and fabricated a catheter that is similar to that described by Schreiber et al. (16,20) but that has been modified for use in studies of chemoprevention. The catheter delivers a predetermined quantity of carcinogen solution and then reabsorbs the carcinogen; the area of carcinogen exposure is limited to a 6-mm length of the trachea 10–16 mm distal to the vocal cords. The use of vital dyes and the development of tumors have confirmed that carcinogen exposure is limited to this area of the trachea.

The influence of various MNU dosing regimens on both the toxic reactions of animals and the incidence of tracheal cancer (table) has been detailed in two publications (17,18) from our laboratory. As a result of these studies, treatment of animals once weekly with a solution of 0.5% MNU appears to be optimal for studies of the inhibition of carcinogenesis. Weekly administration at higher concentrations of MNU (1.0%) was found to be toxic, as was instillation of 0.5% MNU twice a week. Desired cancer incidence levels can be obtained by varying the length of MNU treatment; administration of 0.5% MNU once weekly for 15 weeks yields a cancer incidence of approximately 60% at 6 months, whereas shorter periods of MNU treatment yield fewer cancers. The dose-response curve for MNU-induced tracheal cancer appears to be approximately linear: from 0 to 75% cancer incidence.

Table. Effect of Weekly or Biweekly Instillations of Various Concentrations of MNU on Induction of Tracheal Cancer

Treatment	No. Hamsters	No. Surviving Treatment	% Survival	No. Hamsters with Cancers	% Incidence of Cancers[a]
Once/week					
Vehicle	10	10	100	0	—
MNU, 0.5%	20	19	95	13	68
MNU, 0.25%	20	18	90	6	33
MNU, 0.125%	20	17	85	0	—
Twice/week					
Vehicle	11	8	73	0	—
MNU, 0.5%	15	11	73	11	100
MNU, 0.25%	15	10	67	7	70
MNU, 0.125%	15	14	93	3	21

[a]Includes only those animals that survived the treatment period.
Abbreviation: MNU, N-methyl-N-nitrosourea.

Lung Cancer Model (*N*-nitrosodiethylamine/Syrian Golden Hamster)

The organ-specific carcinogenicity of *N*-nitrosodiethylamine (DEN) for the respiratory tract of Syrian golden hamsters was demonstrated by several studies (11,21,22), including those from our laboratory (23). Regardless of the route of administration of DEN, tumors developed predominantly in the trachea, oral cavity, and larynx with a much lower incidence in the stem bronchi and peripheral lung. The high sensitivity of the trachea to DEN carcinogenesis was shown by Dontenwill (24) using an intrasplenic implantation technique. More recent biochemical studies have shown that tracheal tissue metabolized DEN efficiently and subsequently formed ethylated DNA adducts (25,26). A dose-response correlation for the induction of upper respiratory tract tumors was demonstrated by Montesano and Saffiotti (22) in hamsters injected subcutaneously at dose levels of 0.5, 1, 2, and 4 mg of DEN once weekly for 12 weeks. Depending on the dose level, tumors developed as early as 11 weeks; the incidences ranged from 88–100% in the trachea—mostly papillomas—to 17–75% in the nasal cavities and the larynx. In a total of 142 animals, only three tumors of the lung were observed. The malignant potential of these tumors was demonstrated by transplantation experiments.

The pathogenesis of DEN-induced neoplasms of the respiratory tract was investigated (27,28) by the serial kill of Syrian golden hamsters injected subcutaneously with a high dose of DEN (17.8 mg/kg; 0.1 LD_{50}) twice weekly for 20 weeks (total dose, 72 mg/100 g). When the study was terminated at 24 weeks, this dose schedule yielded a tumor incidence of 90–100% in the trachea and 60–70% in the lung (29). Similar tumor incidence was observed in our studies, which used the same experimental protocol. Serial kill studies by Reznik-Schuller (29) showed that the lung tumors originated primarily from pulmonary clara and endocrine cells, whereas the tracheal tumors were derived from basal cells. Since lung tumors with features of pulmonary endocrine cells (small-cell carcinoma) account for 20–30% of all lung cancers, the DEN hamster model appears to be a suitable system for evaluating potential chemopreventive agents against respiratory tract cancer.

CHEMOPREVENTION: RESPIRATORY CANCER AND RETINOIDS

Most primary human cancers arise in epithelial tissues that depend on retinoids for normal cellular differentiation (30,31). Several epidemiologic investigations have noted an inverse relationship between vitamin A intake and the risk for developing cancer (32–35). Over the past few years, considerable effort has been directed toward the experimental modulation of the tumorigenesis of these epithelia by retinoids; although reports have appeared on the inhibition of carcinogenesis in many epithelial tissues, the majority of these studies have dealt with the chemoprevention of cancers of the skin, mammary gland, and urinary bladder.

The rationale for using retinoids as chemopreventive agents, or inhibitors of carcinogenesis, dates back almost 60 years. As early as 1922, Mori (36) observed that a deficiency of vitamin A led to metaplastic changes in the epithelium of the respiratory tract. The normal ciliated columnar epithelium of the trachea became flattened, lost nuclei, and became cornified, whereas the underlying layer of cells exhibited typical keratohyaline granules. The remarkable observations of Mori on the development of such retinoid-deficient squamous metaplasia indicated a process closely akin to that induced by certain chemical carcinogens (18,37). A more direct link between retinoids and cancer appeared in 1926, when Fujimake (38) observed the development of carcinomas of the stomach of rats maintained on a vitamin A–deficient diet. Other investigators have also shown that animals fed a diet deficient in retinoids and subsequently exposed to chemical carcinogens developed not only a greater than normal incidence of respiratory cancers but also putative precursors to these malignancies (39,40).

In addition to establishing the relationship between retinoid deficiency and neoplasia, other studies have indicated that retinoids can reverse premalignant changes (41,42), suppress malignant transformation (43), and inhibit tumor promotion (44). Several investigators have extended these studies to show that exogenous retinoids can inhibit tumor formation in vivo at several different organ sites.

Saffiotti and co-workers (45) were the first to describe an inhibitory effect of retinoids on respiratory carcinogenesis. However, these studies have been equivocal and, in some cases, contradictory. In the study by Saffiotti et al., tumors were induced in hamsters by the intra-tracheal instillation of benzo[a]pyrene adsorbed onto ferric oxide particles (3 mg benzo[a]pyrene plus 3 mg ferric oxide suspended in 0.2 ml saline) once a week for 10 weeks. Treatment with retinyl palmitate markedly reduced both the incidence and the number of respiratory tumors. Retinyl acetate was ineffective, however, in inhibiting the development of lung tumors induced by the Saffiotti technique. Nettesheim et al. (46), on the other hand, showed that in rats retinyl acetate inhibited metastatic lung nodules induced with 3-methylcholanthrene. A study by Port et al. (47) showed bronchial carcinoma induced by the Saffiotti technique to be effectively inhibited by 13-*cis*–retinoic acid, although enhancement of MNU-induced tra-cheobronchial carcinogenesis has been reported with 13-*cis*–retinoic acid, ethyl retinamide, and *N*-(4-hydroxyethyl)retinamide (48). In an early study, *N*-(4-hydroxyphenyl)retinamide (4-HPR) neither enhanced nor inhibited tracheobronchial carcinogenesis induced with MNU (49). More recently, however, we have found that 4-HPR is an effective inhibitor of DEN-induced lung carcinogenesis in the hamster (Figure 1) but has little effect on MNU-induced tracheobronchial carcinogenesis in this species. As indicated in Figure 1, 4-HPR in combina-tion with selenium and vitamin E was more effective than when these agents were administered alone (50).

A combination of selenium and vitamin E was ineffective in inhibiting tracheal carcino-genesis also, whereas the addition of 4-HPR to this combination of agents effectively inhibited the formation of squamous cell carcinomas of the trachea (Figure 2).

Additional studies (50) showed that both the natural retinoid, retinol, and the carotenoid, β-carotene, which is converted to retinol, are ineffective in suppressing respiratory carcino-genesis induced with either MNU or DEN. However, a combination of retinol and β-carotene inhibited the development of lung adenocarcinoma induced with DEN.

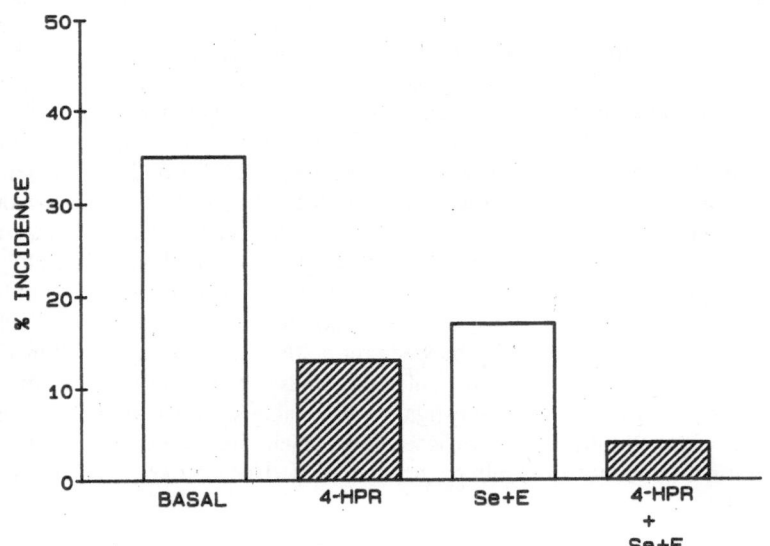

Figure 1. Effect of 4-HPR alone or in com-bination with selenium and vitamin E on inci-dence of lung adeno-squamous carcinomas induced in male ham-sters with diethylnitro-samine. 4-HPR, seleni-um, and vitamin E administered as sup-plements to the basal diet (AIN-76A). Hatched bars are significantly different from basal.

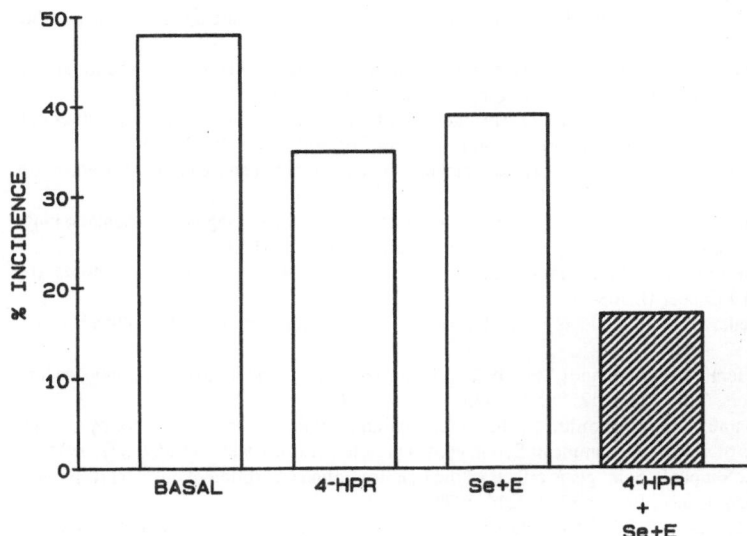

Figure 2. Effect of 4-HPR alone or in combination with selenium and vitamin E on incidence of squamous cell carcinoma of the trachea induced in male hamsters with methylnitrosourea. 4-HPR, selenium, and vitamin E administered as supplements to the basal diet (AIN-76A). Hatched bars are significantly different from basal.

The experiments described demonstrate that some natural and synthetic retinoids are highly effective in inhibiting respiratory carcinogenesis induced with MNU, DEN, or both. It is also apparent that in some cases the synthetic retinoids are more effective than the natural retinoids and are considerably less toxic. In experimental systems that exhibit definite initiation and promotion stages of carcinogenesis (mammary, skin), the retinoids have proved to be highly effective chemopreventive agents. However, when a definitive promotional phase is absent in an experimental tumor system or is ill defined (tracheobronchial, lung), ambiguous results as to the chemopreventive effectiveness of the retinoids have been obtained; in isolated cases, the compounds may even promote carcinogenesis. Nevertheless, the overwhelming evidence indicates that retinoids inhibit carcinogenesis in such experimental tumor systems. Furthermore, the additive or synergistic effect of combinations of agents may prove clinically important to reducing toxicity while increasing efficacy.

ACKNOWLEDGMENTS

The studies conducted in our laboratory were supported in part by NO1-CN-45192-04, NO1-CN-45192-09, NO1-CN-45192-13, and NO1-CN-85097-03 from the National Cancer Institute.

We are greatly indebted to Mrs. Patti Moser for her expert assistance in preparing the manuscript and to our staff for their technical expertise.

REFERENCES

1. Nettesheim P. Respiratory carcinogenesis studies with the Syrian golden hamster: A review. Prog Exp Tumor Res 16:185–200, 1972.
2. Saffiotti U. Experimental respiratory tract carcinogenesis. Prog Exp Tumor Res 11:302–333, 1969.
3. Kuschner M, Laskin S, Cristofano E, Nelson N. Experimental carcinoma of the lung. In Proceedings of the Third National Cancer Conference. Philadelphia: JB Lippincott, 1956, pp. 485–495.
4. Stevenson JL, von Haam E. Induction of pulmonary tumors in C57BL mice using strings impregnated with 20-methylcholanthrene. Acta Cytol 7:126–128, 1963.
5. Lisco H, Finkel MP. Observations on lung pathology following the inhalation of radioactive cerium. Federation Proceedings 8:360, 1949.

6. Kuschner M, Laskin S, Nelson N, Altshuler B. Radiation-induced bronchogenic carcinoma in rats. Am J Pathol 34:554–564, 1958.
7. Harris CC, Kaufman DG, Jackson F, Smith JM, Dedick P, Saffiotti U. Atypical cilia in the tracheobronchial epithelium of the hamster during respiratory carcinogenesis. J Pathol 114:17–19, 1974.
8. Harris CC, Kaufman DG, Sporn MB, Saffiotti U. Histogenesis of squamous metaplasia and squamous cell carcinoma of the respiratory epithelium in an animal model. Cancer Chemother Rep 4:43–54, 1973.
9. Saffiotti U, Cefis F, Kolb LH. A method for the experimental induction of bronchogenic carcinoma. Cancer Res 28:104–124, 1968.
10. Saffiotti U, Cefis F, Kolb LH, Grote MI. Intratracheal injections of particulate carcinogens into hamster lungs (abstract). Proceedings of the American Association for Cancer Research 4:59, 1963.
11. Herrold KM. Effect of route of administration on the carcinogenic action of diethylnitrosamine (N-nitrosodiethylamine). Br J Cancer 18:763–767, 1964.
12. Mohr U, Althoff J, Authaler A. Diaplacental effect of the carcinogen diethylnitrosamine in the golden hamster. Cancer Res 26:2349–2352, 1966.
13. Reznik-Schuller H. Proliferation of endocrine (A pud-type) cells during early N-diethylnitrosamine-induced lung carcinogenesis in hamsters. Cancer Lett 1:255–258, 1976.
14. Spit BJ, Feron VJ. Comparative study of the ultrastructure of tracheal and pulmonary tumours induced by multiple intratracheal instillations of diethylnitrosamine in Syrian golden hamsters. Eur J Cancer 11:867–872, 1975.
15. Stenback FG, Ferrero A, Shubik P. Synergistic effects of diethylnitrosamine and different dusts on respiratory carcinogenesis in hamsters. Cancer Res 33:2209–2214, 1973.
16. Schreiber H, Schreiber K, Martin DH. Experimental tumor induction in a circumscribed region of the hamster trachea: Correlation of histology and exfoliative cytology. J Natl Cancer Inst 54:187–197, 1975.
17. Grubbs CJ, Moon RC, Norikane K, Thompson HJ, Becci PJ. 1-Methyl-1-nitrosourea induction of cancer in a localized area of the Syrian golden hamster trachea. Prog Exp Tumor Res 24:345–355, 1979.
18. Becci PJ, Thompson HJ, Grubbs CJ, Moon RC. Histogenesis and dose dependence of N-methyl-N-nitrosourea-induced carcinoma in a localized area of the hamster trachea. J Natl Cancer Inst 64:1135–1140, 1980.
19. Grubbs CJ, Becci PJ, Thompson HJ, Moon RC. Carcinogenicity of N-methyl-N-nitrosourea and N-ethyl-N-nitrosourea when applied to a localized area of the hamster trachea. J Natl Cancer Inst 66:961–965, 1981.
20. Schreiber H, Nettesheim P. A new method for pulmonary cytology in rats and hamsters. Cancer Res 32:737–745, 1972.
21. Dontenwill W, Mohr U, Zagel M. Uber die unterschiedliche lungen-carcinogene wirkung des diethylnitrosamin bei hamster und ratte. Z Krebsforsch 64:499–502, 1962.
22. Montesano R, Saffiotti U. Carcinogenic response of the respiratory tract of Syrian golden hamsters to different doses of diethylnitrosamine. Cancer Res 28:2198–2210, 1968.
23. Henry MC, Port CD. Contract No. NIH-NCI-E-69-2148 (IITRI Project No. L06056-13). Annual Report, April 1972–January 1973.
24. Dontenwill W. Experimentelle untersuchungen zur genese des lungen carcinomas. Arzneimittel-Forsch 14:774–780, 1964.
25. Becker RA, Shank RC. Kinetics of formation and persistence of ethylguanines in DNA of rats and hamsters treated with diethylnitrosamine. Cancer Res 45:2076–2084, 1985.
26. Fong AT, Rasmussen RE. DNA ethylation in hamster tissues during subchronic diethylnitrosamine administration and in the hamster trachea after acute diethylnitrosamine administration. Carcinogenesis 7:1457–1461, 1986.
27. Reznik-Schuller H, Reznik G. Experimental pulmonary carcinogenesis. Int Rev Exp Pathol 20:211–281, 1979.
28. Reznik-Schuller H. Pathogenesis of diethylnitrosamine-induced tumors in the Syrian golden hamster trachea. Pathol Res Pract 168:185–192, 1980.
29. Schuller HM, McMahon JB. Inhibition of N-nitrosodiethylamine-induced respiratory tract carcinogenesis by piperonylbutoxide in hamsters. Cancer Res 45:2807–2812, 1985.
30. Wolbach SD, Howe PR. Tissue changes following deprivation of fat-soluble A vitamin. J Exp Med 42:753–778, 1925.
31. Moore T. Vitamin A. Amsterdam: Elsevier Publishing, 1957.
32. Bjelke E. Dietary vitamin A and human lung cancer. Int J Cancer 15:561–565, 1975.
33. Mettlin C, Graham S, Swanson M. Vitamin A and lung cancer. J Natl Cancer Inst 62:1435–1438, 1979.
34. Mettlin C, Graham S. Dietary risk factors in human bladder cancer. Am J Epidemiol 110:255–263, 1979.
35. Hirayama T. Diet and cancer. Nutr Cancer 1:67–81, 1979.
36. Mori S. The changes in the paraocular glands which follow the administration of diets low in fat-soluble A with notes of the effect of the same diets on the salivary glands and the mucosa of the larynx and trachea. Johns Hopkins Hospital Bulletin 33:357–359, 1922.
37. Harris CC, Sporn MB, Kaufman DG. Histogenesis of squamous metaplasias in the hamster tracheal epithelium caused by vitamin A deficiency or benzo[a]pyrene ferric oxide. J Natl Cancer Inst 48:743–761, 1972.
38. Fujimake Y. Formation of gastric carcinoma in albino rats fed on deficient diets. Journal of Cancer Research 10:469–477, 1926.

39. Nettesheim P, Williams ML. The influence of vitamin A on the susceptibility of the rat lung to 3-methylcholanthrene. Int J Cancer 17:351–357, 1976.

40. Smith DM, Rogers AE, Newberne PM. Vitamin A and benzo[a]pyrene carcinogenesis in the respiratory tract of hamsters fed a semisynthetic diet. Cancer Res 35:1485–1488, 1975.

41. Lasnitzki I. Reversal of methylcholanthrene-induced changes in mouse prostates *in vitro* by retinoic acid and its analogues. Br J Cancer 34:239–248, 1976.

42. Lasnitzki I, Goodman DS. Inhibition of the effects of methylcholanthrene on mouse prostate in organ culture by vitamin A and its analogues. Cancer Res 34:1564–1571, 1974.

43. Chopra DP, Wilkoff CJ. Inhibition and reversal by β-retinoic acid of hyperplasia induced in cultured mouse prostate tissue by 3-methylcholanthrene or N-methyl-N-nitro-N-nitrosoguanidine. J Natl Cancer Inst 56:583–589, 1976.

44. Verma AK, Boutwell RK. Vitamin A acid (retinoic acid), a potent inhibitor of 12-O-tetradecanoyl-phorbol-13-acetate-induced ornithine decarboxylase activity in mouse epidermis. Cancer Res 37:2196–2201, 1977.

45. Saffiotti U, Montesano R, Sellakumar AR, Borg SA. Experimental cancer of the lung. Inhibition by vitamin A of the induction of tracheobronchial squamous metaplasia and squamous cell tumors. Cancer 20:857–864, 1967.

46. Nettesheim P, Cone MW, Snyder C. The influence of vitamin A on the susceptibility of the rat lung to 3-methylcholanthrene. Int J Cancer 17:341–357, 1976.

47. Port CD, Sporn MB, Kaufman DG. Prevention of lung cancer in hamsters by 13-cis-retinoic acid (abstract). Proceedings of the American Association for Cancer Research 16:21, 1975.

48. Stinson SP, Reznik G, Donahoe R. Effect of three retinoids on tracheal carcinogenesis with N-methyl-N-nitrosourea in hamsters. J Natl Cancer Inst 66:947–951, 1981.

49. Grubbs CJ, Becci PJ, Moon RC. Characterization of 1-methyl-1-nitrosourea (MNU)-induced tracheal carcinogenesis and the effect of feeding the retinoid N-(4-hydroxyphenyl)retinamide (4-HPR) (abstract). Proceedings of the American Association for Cancer Research 21:102, 1980.

50. Mehta RG, Rao KVN, Detrisac CJ, Kelloff GJ, Moon RC. Inhibition of diethylnitrosamine-induced lung carcinogenesis by retinoids (abstract). Proceedings of the American Association for Cancer Research 29:129, 1988.

The Hamster Cheek Pouch Model of Carcinogenesis and Chemoprevention

Irma B. Gimenez-Conti and Thomas J. Slaga

The University of Texas M. D. Anderson Cancer Center
Science Park—Research Division
Smithville, Texas

The Syrian golden hamster cheek pouch carcinogenesis model is probably the best-known animal system for studying events involved in the development of premalignancy and malignancy in human oral cancer. Like the mouse skin model of carcinogenesis, the hamster cheek pouch model provides data on the effect of carcinogens, promoters, and chemopreventive agents, which makes both these models very useful in selecting chemopreventive agents for human cancer intervention studies (1–8). Our first approach to understanding the important early events that occur in the hamster cheek pouch model of carcinogenesis was to compare this model with the mouse skin model, in which a number of critical events have already been well characterized (9–11). The carcinogenesis studies in the hamster cheek pouch were carried out using multiple applications of 7,12-dimethylbenz[a]anthracene (DMBA) (0.5% in mineral oil, 3 times a week). This protocol induced a hyperplastic response in the pouch epithelium after only a few applications, followed by the appearance after 6–8 weeks of treatment of a variety of dysplastic lesions resembling human premalignant lesions. Benign and malignant tumors (papillomas and squamous cell carcinomas [SCCs]) started to develop after 10 weeks of treatment (12,13).

Probably the best-characterized event that occurs in the hamster cheek pouch during carcinogenesis is the induction of γ-glutamyltranspeptidase (GGT), an enzyme not normally expressed in the hamster cheek pouch. Solt and Shklar (14,15) showed that individual GGT-positive cells or doublet cells are detected histochemically as early as 3 days after the first DMBA treatment. GGT activity has also been demonstrated histochemically in dysplastic areas, papillomas, and well-differentiated SCCs. Unlike in mouse skin, in which the GGT expression seems to be a late event, small foci can be detected at a very early stage (9,13,16) in hamster cheek pouch carcinogenesis.

Changes in the patterns of keratin expression have also been observed in the hamster cheek pouch epithelium during DMBA carcinogenesis (17,18). We have explored the expression of keratins using immunostaining with monospecific antibodies developed by Roop et al. (19) and also a technique that allows immunoblotting analysis of paraffin-embedded tissues (13).

The keratins assayed were K1 (Mr 67,000), K13 (Mr 47,000), and K14 (Mr 55,000). The normal hamster cheek pouch epithelium expressed K14 in the basal layer and K13 in the suprabasal and differentiated layers, whereas K1 was not detected by either immunohisto-chemistry or immunoblotting. Concomitant with DMBA-induced hyperplasia, there were

The Biology and Prevention of Aerodigestive Tract Cancers
Edited by G.R.Newell and W.K. Hong, Plenum Press, New York, 1992

63

some topographic alterations in the distribution of K14. In this case, K14 was no longer restricted to the basal layer, but was also expressed in differentiated cells. The same pattern was also observed in dysplastic lesions and in SCCs. These patterns have been previously described in mouse papillomas, in which immunohistochemistry and in situ hybridization showed that K14 expression is not shut off as epidermal cells move to more superficial layers of the epithelium. It has been speculated that this phenomenon is related to the lack of response to differentiation signals by the genetically altered (initiated) keratinocyte (20). Expression of the K13 differentiation-associated keratin was preserved in this hyperplastic epithelium during all the stages of carcinogenesis, including development of either anaplastic or differentiated lesions.

After 2 weeks of DMBA treatment, K1 expression started as a weak, patchy pattern in suprabasal cells, becoming stronger and more homogeneous at 8 and 16 weeks of treatment. However, K1 was almost absent in SCC, where only small, very well-differentiated areas were stained. We also observed GGT-positive foci in earlier stages of carcinogenesis concomitant with the expression of the K1 keratin. However, it was not possible to find a perfect topographic correspondence between the two events.

Whether the presence of K1 in the pouch epithelium is a simple consequence of hyperplasia or a specific event of DMBA carcinogenic events remains to be elucidated. That human oral and lung premalignant lesions express this type of keratin (21) suggests that such lesions may constitute a necessary step in the pathway to the development of SCC. Although K1 was present in most dysplastic stages, it was essentially absent in the SCC stage, with the exception of small, well-differentiated areas of the tumors. Conversely, K13 did not seem to be affected by malignant transformation and was strongly expressed in the SCC stage (Table 1).

Alterations in the pattern of keratins appeared to be a common feature in the development of SCC in different systems. These alterations probably reflect abnormal differentiation patterns and are excellent tools for monitoring the process of carcinogenesis.

Table 1. Keratins and GGT in Hamster Cheek Pouch During Chemical Carcinogenesis

	Histology	K14	K1	K13	GGT
Skin control (hamster)	Squamous epithelium	++ (Basal)	++	−	−
Cheek pouch					
Control	Squamous epithelium	++ (Basal)	−	+	−
DMBA × 4 wks	Hyperplasia	+++ (All layers)	+ (Patched)	++	+ (Small foci)
DMBA × 8 wks	Hyperplasia with dysplastic areas (premalignant lesion)	+++ (All layers)	+++ (Suprabasal)	++	++ (Large foci)
DMBA × 16 wks	Hyperplasia, premalignant lesions and SCC	+++ (All layers)	− to +++ (Suprabasal)	++	++ (Large foci)
Squamous cell carcinoma	Mostly well-differentiated SCC	+++ (All tumor cells)	+ or − (Small foci)	++	++ (Intratumoral foci)

Abbreviations: GGT, γ-glutamyltranspeptidase; DMBA, 7,12-dimethylbenz[a]anthracene; SCC, squamous cell carcinoma.

Epidermal growth factor (EGF) receptor and transglutaminase type I expression, polyamine (putrescine, spermidine, and spermine) levels, ornithine decarboxylase (ODC) activity, and micronuclei incidence were studied during the carcinogenic process in the hamster model by Shin et al. (22). EGF receptor was not expressed in the normal epithelium, but was present in the hyperplastic epithelium. Stronger staining was observed in both dysplastic areas and SCC, thus suggesting that altered expression of EGF receptor may play an important role in transformation of epithelium from normal, through premalignant changes, to SCC. In normal epithelium of the hamster cheek pouch, transglutaminase I was weakly stained in the spinous layer beneath the keratin layer. After 4 weeks of treatment with DMBA, increased staining was observed mostly in the hyperplastic epithelium. Dysplastic areas and SCC also showed markedly enhanced staining. The more extensive expression of transglutaminase I is similar to the results reported during epidermal hyperplasia in other systems (23,24). Putrescine and spermidine levels and ODC activity increased dramatically in dysplastic epithelium as well as in SCC (25). Micronucleated cells increased after a few weeks of DMBA treatment, and this increase was maintained during all stages of carcinogenesis (Table 2).

TWO-STAGE CARCINOGENESIS PROTOCOL

To develop a two-stage carcinogenesis protocol in the hamster cheek pouch model, we performed a series of short-term experiments using two well-known mouse skin promoters, 12-O-tetradecanoylphorbol-13-acetate (TPA) and benzoyl peroxide (BzPo) (26–28). A number of markers that have been shown to correlate well with the promotion effect of a compound were studied, as well as different solvents, doses, and times of administration. Table 3 summarizes the results of the expression of K1, nucleolar organizer regions (NORs), and hyperplasia in hamster cheek pouch after treatment with TPA or BzPo in acetone solvent. Changes in NOR activity in this model have been demonstrated using a silver-colloid technique (29,30). When mineral oil, the more common vehicle in this model, was used as the solvent of TPA and BzPo in both the mouse skin and the hamster cheek pouch models, the induction of hyperplasia was less pronounced than when acetone was used (Table 4). Unlike in the mouse skin model, BzPo was a better inducer of short-term markers of tumor promotion

Table 2. Hamster Cheek Pouch Carcinogenesis Model Changes with Time after DMBA Treatment

	Weeks			
	0	1–4	8	16
Hyperplasia	–	+++	+++	++++
GGT	–	+	++	++
Ornithine decarboxylase and polyamines	+	++	+++	+++++
Transglutaminase I	+	++	+++	++++
EGF receptor	–	+	++	++
Micronuclei	–	++	++	++
Leukoplakia	–	–	++	+
Dysplasia	–	–	++	+++
Squamous cell carcinoma	–	–	–	+

Abbreviations: DMBA, 7,12-dimethylbenz[a]anthracene; GGT, γ-glutamyltranspeptidase; EGF, epidermal growth factor.

Table 3. Effect of TPA and Benzoyl Peroxide in the Hamster Cheek Pouch (Acetone Solvent)

Promoter	Hours After Last Treatment	Hyperplasia (μm)	% NOR of High Activity	K1
Control		23.56	9.1	–
TPA (200 μg) [2 × /2 wks]	24	33.64	15	+—
	48	34.73	11.05	+—
Benzoyl peroxide (40 mg) [3 × /2 wks]	24	54.27	27.32	++—
	48	63.53	24.87	++—

Abbreviations: TPA, 12-O-tetradecanoylphorbol-13-acetate; NOR, nucleolar organizer region.

Table 4. Effect of TPA in the Hamster Cheek Pouch (Mineral Oil Solvent)

Promoter	Epithelial Thickness (μm)		
	24 hr	48 hr	72 hr
Control (mineral oil alone)	31.33	31.33	31.33
Single application dose of TPA			
2 μg	32.64	—	—
10 μg	32.83	29.70	31.11
50 μg	32.97	29.84	32.37
100 μg	35.10	39.18	33.19
Multiple application (4 × /2 wks)			
100 μg	36.78	35.29	—

Abbreviation: TPA, 12-O-tetradecanoylphorbol-13-acetate.

CONCLUSION

The hamster cheek pouch carcinogenesis system is an excellent model for studying carcinogenic mechanisms as well as for investigating approaches to chemoprevention and chemointervention. In the last few years, cellular and molecular mechanisms of carcinogenesis in this model have begun to be understood, and several markers of carcinogenesis have been described. These studies will contribute to more efficient protocols for assaying chemopreventive agents. Furthermore, work is under way in this model to define a two-stage carcinogenesis protocol (initiation/promotion) that will allow studies on the effect of chemopreventive agents at the initiation or promotion phase of carcinogenesis, or both.

Future studies using this model will be aimed at a better understanding of the molecular changes that occur during carcinogenesis. This knowledge will hopefully provide an expanded rationale for pursuing new chemopreventive approaches.

REFERENCES

1. Solt DB, Polverini PP, Calderon L. Carcinogenic response of hamster buccal pouch epithelium to 4 polycyclic aromatin hydrocarbons. J Oral Pathol 16:294–302, 1987.
2. Odukoya O, Shklar G. Initiation and promotion in experimental oral carcinogenesis. Oral Surg Oral Med Oral Pathol 58:315–320, 1984.
3. Odukoya O, Hawach F, Shklar G. Retardation of experimental oral cancer by topical vitamin E. Nutr Cancer 6:98–104, 1984.

4. Trickler D, Shklar G. Prevention by vitamin E of experimental oral carcinogenesis. J Natl Cancer Inst 78:165–169, 1987.
5. Shklar G, Schwartz J, Grau D, Trickler DP, Wallace KD. Inhibition of hamster buccal pouch carcinogenesis by 13-*cis*-retinoic acid. Oral Surg 50:45–52, 1980.
6. Schwartz J, Shklar G. Regression of experimental oral carcinomas by local injection of β-carotene and canthaxanthin. Nutr Cancer 11:35–40, 1988.
7. Schwartz J, Shklar G. Regression of experimental hamster cancer by beta carotene and algae extracts. J Oral Maxillofac Surg 45:510–515, 1987.
8. Messadi DV, Billings P, Shklar G, Kennedy AR. Inhibition of oral carcinogenesis by a protease inhibitor. J Natl Cancer Inst 76:447–452, 1986.
9. Aldaz CM, Conti CJ, Larcher F, Trono D, Roop DR, Chesner J, Whitehead T, Slaga TJ. Sequential development of aneuploidy, keratin modifications, an γ-glutamyltransferase expression in mouse skin papillomas. Cancer Res 48:3253–3257, 1988.
10. Gimenez-Conti IB, Aldaz CM, Bianchi AB, Roop DR, Slaga TJ, Conti CJ. Early expression of type I K13 keratin in the progression of mouse skin papillomas. Carcinogenesis 11:1995–1999, 1990.
11. Bianchi AB, Aldaz CM, Conti CJ. Non-random duplication of the chromosome bearing a mutated Ha-ras-1 allele in mouse skin tumors. Proc Natl Acad Sci USA 87:6902–6906, 1990.
12. Morris AL. Factors influencing experimental carcinogenesis in the hamster cheek pouch. J Dent Res 40:3–15, 1961.
13. Gimenez-Conti IB, Shin DM, Bianchi AB, Roop DR, Hong WK, Conti CJ, Slaga TJ. Changes in keratin expression during 7,12-dimethylbenz[a]anthracene-induced hamster cheek pouch carcinogenesis. Cancer Res 50:4441–4445, 1990.
14. Solt DB. Localization of gamma-glutamyl transpeptidase in hamster buccal pouch epithelium treated with 7,12-dimethylbenz[a]anthracene. J Natl Cancer Inst 67:193–199, 1981.
15. Solt DB, Shklar G. Rapid induction of γ-glutamyltranspeptidase-rich intraepithelial clones in 7,12-dimethylbenz[a]anthracene-treated hamster buccal pouch. Cancer Res 42:285–291, 1982.
16. Odajima T, Solt DB, Calderon SL. Persistence of γ-glutamyltranspeptidase-positive foci during hamster buccal pouch carcinogenesis. Cancer Res 44:2062–2067, 1984.
17. Murase N, Fukui S, Mori M. Heterogeneity of keratin distribution in the oral mucosa and skin of mammals as determined using monoclonal antibodies. Histochemistry 85:265–276, 1986.
18. Tatemoto Y, Fukui S, Oosumi H, Horike H, Mori M. Expression of keratins during experimentally induced carcinogenesis in hamster cheek pouch visualized polyclonal and monoclonal antibodies. Histochemistry 86:445–452, 1987.
19. Roop DR, Cheng CK, Titterington L, Meyers CA, Stanley JR, Steinert PM, Yuspa SH. Synthetic peptides corresponding to keratin subunits elicit highly specific antibodies. J Biol Chem 6259:8037–8040, 1984.
20. Roop DR, Kreig TM, Mehrel T, Cheng CK, Yuspa SH. Transcriptional control of high molecular weight keratin gene expression in multistage skin carcinogenesis. Cancer Res 48:3245–3252, 1988.
21. Moll R, Franke WW, Schiller B, Geiger B, Krepler R. The catalog of human cytokeratins: Patterns of expression in normal epithelia, tumors and cultured cells. Cell 31:11–24, 1982.
22. Shin DM, Gimenez IB, Lee JS, Nishioka K, Wargovich MJ, Thacher S, Lotan R, Slaga TJ, Hong WK. Expression of epidermal growth factor receptor, polyamine levels, ornithine decarboxylase activity, micronuclei and transglutaminase I in a 7,12-dimethylbenz[a]anthracene-induced hamster buccal pouch carcinogenesis model. Cancer Res 50:2505–2510, 1990.
23. Thacher SM. Purification of keratinocyte transglutaminase and its expression during squamous differentiation. J Invest Dermatol 89:578–584, 1989.
24. Mansbridges JN, Knapp AM. Changes in keratinocyte maturation during wound healing. J Invest Dermatol 89:253–263, 1987.
25. O'Brien TG. The induction of ornithine decarboxylase as an early possible obligatory event in mouse skin carcinogenesis. Cancer Res 36:2644–2653, 1976.
26. Klein-Szanto AJP, Major SM, Slaga TJ. Induction of dark keratinocytes by 12-O-tetradecanoylphorbol-13-acetate and mezerein as an indicator of tumor-promoting efficiency. Carcinogenesis 1:399–406, 1980.
27. Slaga TJ, Klein-Szanto AJP, Triplett LL, Yotti LP, Trosko JE. Skin tumor promoting activity of benzoyl peroxide, a widely used free radical-generating compound. Science 213:1023–1025, 1981.
28. Klein-Szanto AJP, Slaga TJ. Effects of peroxides on rodent skin: Epidermal hyperplasia and tumor promotion. J Invest Dermatol 79:30–34, 1982.
29. Ploton D, Menager M, Jeannesson P, Himber G, Pigeon F, Adnet JJ. Improvement in the staining and in the visualization of the argyrophilic proteins of the nucleolar organizer region at the optical level. Histochem J 18:5–14, 1986.
30. Yoshimi N, Gimenez-Conti I, Conti CJ, Slaga TJ. Changes of nucleolar organizer regions (NORs) in hamster cheek pouch chemical carcinogenesis. Proceedings of the American Association for Cancer Research 31:125, 1990.

Culture Conditions Affect Expression of the $\alpha^6\beta_4$ Integrin Associated with Aggressive Behavior in Head and Neck Cancer

Thomas E. Carey, Leena Laurikainen, Angelika Ptok,
Timothy Reinke, Keith Linder, Thankam S. Nair,
and Cynthia Marcelo[1]

Laboratory of Head and Neck Cancer Biology
Department of Otolaryngology, Head and Neck Surgery
Division of Head and Neck Oncology
Research Division of the [1] Department of Dermatology
University of Michigan Cancer Center
Ann Arbor, Michigan

INTRODUCTION

Prevention of disease has always been more effective than treatment. Sanitation practices and vaccines have eliminated many of the most dreaded and lethal diseases of man and domestic animals. Cancer, a devastating disease caused by unregulated growth of genetically altered cells, is as daunting a challenge today as smallpox was in Edward Jenner's time two centuries ago. Fortunately, we are on the threshold of a new era in biology. We can now examine growth-regulatory mechanisms at the cellular and molecular levels, and we can begin to apply what we learn in new clinical and experimental systems.

Chemoprevention of cancer is one product of this type of study, but as has happened so often in the past, remarkable clinical techniques have been developed before we have fully understood their molecular basis. The demonstration by Dr. W.K. Hong and his colleagues (1) that retinoic acid can decrease the rate of second primary cancers in patients with head and neck cancer is a milestone in cancer biology and an example of this phenomenon. In spite of this preliminary but dramatic clinical success, we know relatively little about the mechanisms at the cellular level that are responsible for this effect of retinoic acid.

My charge today is to discuss cultured epithelial cells and their possible use for in vitro mechanisms important in chemoprevention. Although our laboratory at the University of Michigan Cancer Center (Ann Arbor) is not directly involved in chemoprevention, we are investigating factors that affect expression of cell surface structures linked to growth and differentiation of normal cells and to tumor progression in malignant cells. Since chemopreventive compounds may act through the regulation of cell differentiation (2,3), the model systems we employ may be useful for the study of this class of agents.

The Biology and Prevention of Aerodigestive Tract Cancers
Edited by G.R.Newell and W.K. Hong, Plenum Press, New York, 1992

69

I will present preliminary research findings from the epithelial culture systems we used to identify antigenic markers that are associated with tumor behavior. These consist of an in vitro human model of squamous cell carcinoma (SCC) cell lines and normal keratinocytes grown under culture conditions that regulate the differentiation of normal but not malignant cells. We have also just begun using an in vitro/in vivo animal model system derived from the rabbit VX2 squamous carcinoma that may prove very helpful for future studies.

We previously reported that the A9 antigen (defined by monoclonal antibody UM-A9) is expressed differently on normal and malignant cells growing in culture and that the A9 antigen is also expressed differently on primary and recurrent or metastatic tumors from the same patients (4). Subsequently, we showed that the intensity of expression of A9 in tumor sections was an indicator of early recurrence in patients with head and neck SCC (5). These results suggest that the A9 antigen has a functional role in tumor behavior. We recently demonstrated that the A9 antigen is a heterodimer of two glycosylated polypeptide chains that have the same immunologic and biochemical properties as the $\alpha^6\beta_4$ epithelial integrin (6), a member of the integrin family of extracellular matrix receptors (7). The mechanisms that cause altered expression of this integrin in malignant cells are not known. If, as we expect from our accumulated data, this marker is functionally associated with aggressive tumor behavior, then its regulation might be an appropriate target of chemoprevention strategies. I will present some preliminary experiments in which we have begun to examine the factors that control expression of the A9/$\alpha^6\beta_4$ integrin in squamous epithelial cells.

MATERIALS AND METHODS

Cell Culture

Squamous carcinoma cells UM-SCC-10B, 14C, and 38 were established in our laboratory from carcinomas of the larynx (10B) and oral cavity (14C, 38), and UM-MEL-1 was established from a malignant melanoma of the skin as described previously by Kimmel and Carey (4). Tumor cell lines were cultured in M10 medium consisting of Dulbecco's modified Eagle's medium supplemented with 2 mM L-glutamine, nonessential amino acids (components purchased from Sigma Chemical Company, St. Louis, MO), and 10% fetal bovine serum (Hyclone Laboratories Inc., Logan, UT). Tumor cells were used during midlogarithmic growth unless described otherwise. Subconfluent cultures were harvested with recrystallized porcine trypsin (0.1% w/v) (Sigma) and 2 mM ethylenediaminetetraacetic acid (EDTA) in Puck's saline A.

Normal keratinocytes were cultivated from normal adult skin obtained during elective reduction mammaplasties or from neonatal foreskins using adaptations of the method of Boyce and Ham (8). In brief, the skin samples were trimmed of fat and subdermal components, minced into small pieces, incubated overnight at 37°C in collagenase A (2 mg/ml) (Sigma), and split into dermal and epidermal halves. The keratinocytes were released from the epidermal component by digestion with trypsin-EDTA for 20 minutes at room temperature. After neutralization of the trypsin with M10 or soybean trypsin inhibitor, the keratinocytes were washed and resuspended in keratinocyte medium (KM) consisting of MCDB 153 (8) containing 0.09 mM calcium, 50 µg/ml bovine pituitary extract and 2–5 ng/ml epidermal growth factor (EGF); then they were plated in flasks and incubated at 37°C in a humidified atmosphere containing 5% CO_2.

Antibodies

UM-A9 was developed in our laboratory (4) and was shown to identify the $\alpha^6\beta_4$ integrin by immunoprecipitation and preclearing experiments (6). Hybridoma supernatants from a

70

standardized batch of supernatant were used throughout. Hybridoma supernatant containing GoH3, a rat anti-α^6 monoclonal antibody (9), was generously provided by Dr. A. Sonnenberg (University of Amsterdam, The Netherlands).

Immunofluorescence Assays

For immunofluorescence assays of cells in monolayers, the cells were plated on glass coverslips in plastic culture dishes. For observing cells in suspension, tumor cells and keratinocytes were harvested by brief trypsin-EDTA exposure. To examine antigen expression under conditions that prevent normal keratinocyte differentiation, the cells were grown in keratinocyte growth medium and were fed every 2 days. To examine antigen expression under conditions that induce differentiation of normal keratinocytes, cells were fed with M10 or with keratinocyte growth medium containing a high level of calcium (1.0 mM).

Cells were washed with phosphate-buffered saline (PBS), incubated with normal goat serum, washed again, and incubated at 4°C for 2 hours with either UM-A9 hybridoma supernatant, GoH3 rat hybridoma supernatant, or isotype-matched, control, hybridoma supernatants (1B2/B5, a murine IgG_{2a}; and AIIB2, a rat IgG, provided by Drs. Mark Kaminski [University of Michigan, Ann Arbor] and Carolyn Damsky [University of California, San Francisco], respectively). The cells were washed again and were incubated with fluorescein or rhodamine-conjugated goat anti-mouse or anti-rat IgG for 1 hour at 4°C. After final washings, the cells were fixed with ice-cold acetone for 3 minutes, coverslips were mounted, and the cells were examined under the fluorescence microscope. In some experiments, the cells were first harvested with trypsin-EDTA and then washed and stained in suspension as described above.

Northern Blotting

RNA was isolated from logarithmically growing cells by a modification of the guanidinium thiocyanate procedure (10). Cells were washed with ice-cold PBS, placed on ice, and lysed directly in the culture dish with 4 M guanidinium thiocyanate containing 25 mM Na citrate, pH 7.0, 0.5% sarcosyl, and 0.1 M 2-mercaptoethanol. The mixture was extracted with phenol:chloroform:isoamylalcohol and centrifuged at $10,000 \times g$. RNA was precipitated from the aqueous phase with isopropanol, washed with 75% ethanol, air dried, redissolved in water treated with diethylpyrocarbonate, and stored at $-70°C$. RNA concentration was determined by absorbance at 260 nm and analyzed for β_4 and α^6 message by northern analysis.

RNA (10 µg/lane) was electrophoresed in 1.2% agarose-formaldehyde gels, stained with ethidium bromide, photographed, and transferred to nylon membranes as described by Sambrook et al. (11). Membranes were prehybridized at 42°C in formamide with denatured salmon sperm DNA, hybridized at the same temperature with ^{32}P-labeled probes, washed, and autoradiographed. RNA loading was assessed by hybridization to cyclophilin, which has constant expression in normal keratinocytes (12).

Plasmid DNA containing a 3.8-kb *Eco*RI fragment for the β_4 chain (cDNA clone P.6.3) (13) was provided by Martin Hemler (Dana-Farber Cancer Institute, Boston); clone K163 for β_4 (14) and clone 1363 for α^6 (Hogervorst F et al., 1991, unpublished data) were provided by Dr. A. Sonnenberg. The cyclophilin probe was provided by Dr. Brian Nickoloff (University of Michigan, Ann Arbor) with permission from Dr. Matt Harding (Vertex Pharmaceuticals, Cambridge, MA). Plasmid DNA was extracted from transformed *Escherichia coli* by alkaline lysis (16), purified by polyethylene glycol precipitation (11), digested with *Eco*RI (according to the manufacturer's instructions), isolated by electrophoresis in 1% low-melt agarose, dissolved in distilled water, and labeled by the random primer method described by Feinberg and Vogelstein (17).

RESULTS

$\alpha^6\beta_4$ Integrin mRNA Expression in Normal Keratinocytes and Tumor Cells

Messenger RNA samples extracted from logarithmically growing normal keratinocytes and UM-SCC-38 cells, derived from a highly malignant SCC of the oral cavity, were compared for expression of β_4 and α^6 message. Because UM-SCC-38 was known to be a high expressor of the $\alpha^6\beta_4$ integrin, we expected the tumor cells to express higher message levels than normal cells. However, as shown in Figure 1, the normal keratinocytes had higher message levels even though an equal amount of RNA was loaded in each lane. Our first thought was that since the tumor cells were grown in M10 and the keratinocytes were grown in KM, the EGF in the KM was responsible for stimulating β_4 expression in the normal cells. To test this possibility, keratinocytes and UM-SCC-38 cells were each grown in KM, in KM+ (KM supplemented with $2 \times$ EGF), and in KM– (KM without EGF). The level of β_4 expression increased in the

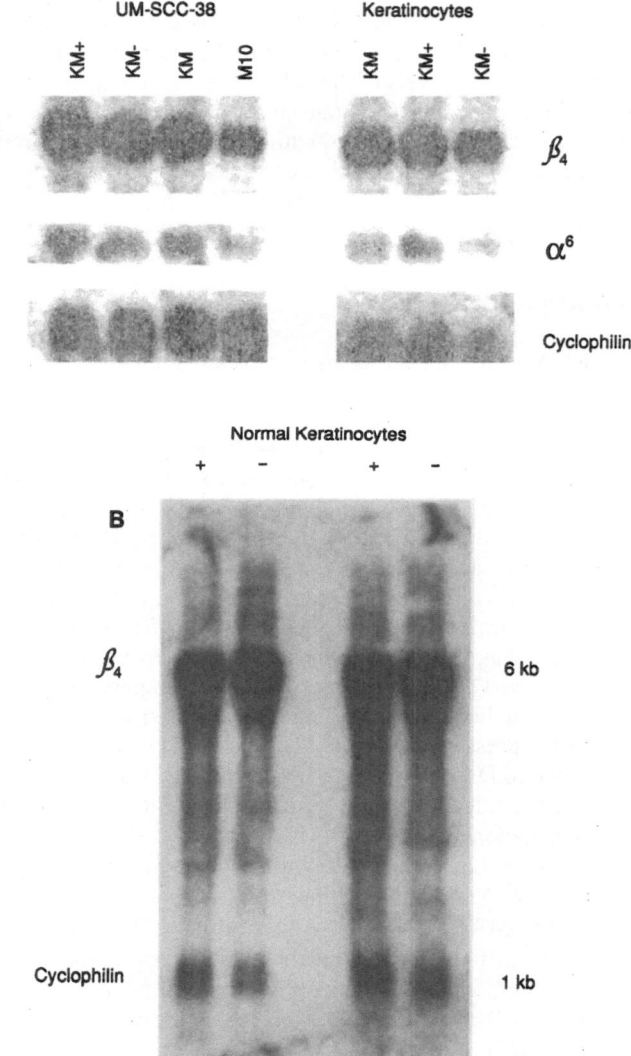

Figure 1. Northern analysis of α^6 and β_4 mRNA expression in normal and malignant keratinocytes. Cells were grown either in Dulbecco's modified Eagle's medium with 10% fetal bovine serum (M10) or in serum-free keratinocyte medium (KM) containing epidermal growth factor (EGF) (2–5 ng/ml) and low calcium (0.09 mM). In some cases (indicated by KM+), double EGF (4–10 ng/ml) was added to the keratinocyte medium. In other cases, no EGF was added (KM–). (A) The blot was probed first with β_4, revealing a band of approximately 6 kb; it was stripped and autoradiographed to ensure that no signal remained and then reprobed with α^6 and cyclophilin, revealing bands of approximately 6 and 1 kb, respectively; (B) To confirm that EGF did not affect β_4 expression in normal keratinocytes, the experiment was repeated on another blot and probed simultaneously with β_4 and cyclophilin. + indicates EGF was added to KM; – indicates no EGF was added.

UM-SCC-38 cells grown in KM, but there appeared to be no effect of EGF on β_4 expression in either the tumor cells or the normal keratinocytes (Figure 1A). The experiment was repeated with normal keratinocytes grown in KM+ or KM– to confirm this result (Figure 1B). The blot from Figure 1A was stripped and reprobed with the α^6 and the cyclophilin probes. The cyclophilin hybridization showed that equal amounts of RNA were loaded in each lane. As before, the lowest level of integrin message expression was found in the UM-SCC-38 cells grown in M10. There seemed to be no effect of EGF on the level of α^6 expression in the UM-SCC-38 cells. EGF may have had some effect on α^6 expression in the normal keratinocytes since the lanes loaded with RNA from cells grown in KM (2–5 ng/ml EGF) and KM+ (4–10 ng/ml EGF) showed stronger hybridization signals than did the RNA from cells grown in KM–, a medium lacking EGF.

To determine whether this finding was unique to UM-SCC-38, we repeated the experiment using UM-SCC-10B, another strong A9/$\alpha^6\beta_4$ antigen expressor. RNA was prepared from UM-SCC-10B and UM-MEL-1 melanoma cells (negative for A9/$\alpha^6\beta_4$ antigen expression), both grown in M10 and KM; from UM-SCC-38 cells grown in M10; and from keratinocytes grown in KM as controls. As shown in Figure 2, the highest level of expression was observed in the normal keratinocytes grown in KM. As expected, no β_4 expression was detected in the melanoma cells regardless of the culture conditions; in UM-SCC-10B cells grown in M10, β_4 mRNA was very low. But, just as we had observed with UM-SCC-38, β_4 expression was elevated in KM.

A9/$\alpha^6\beta_4$ Expression in Malignant Keratinocytes in KM and M10

To determine how A9/$\alpha^6\beta_4$ antigen expression in tumor cells corresponded to the effects we observed on message levels, we selected another high A9/$\alpha^6\beta_4$ expressor tumor cell line, UM-SCC-14C. Cells of this line expressed very high levels of the A9/$\alpha^6\beta_4$ antigen as determined by flow cytometry; the highest we have observed thus far. A cell suspension harvested from a culture fed with M10 and stained with the UM-A9 antibody for flow cytometry is shown in Figure 3. We grew these cells on coverslips for 3 days in either KM or M10 and examined them in situ for A9/$\alpha^6\beta_4$ expression by immunofluorescence. The results are shown in Figure 4. In KM (Figure 4A), the integrin expression was distributed along numerous fingerlike projections and pseudopodia. Similar results were observed in normal keratinocytes; in addition, the longer the cells were on a coverslip, the more covered the surface became with "footprints" of fluorescently stained antigen (not shown). By contrast, the cell morphology in M10 (Figure 4B) was more epithelioid. The cells formed into monolayers, and the antigen expression was distributed at cell–cell junctions and at the edges of the cells.

$\alpha^6\beta_4$ Expression in Normal Keratinocytes Grown to Confluence in KM and M10

To determine if the change in the A9/$\alpha^6\beta_4$ expression pattern was a result of cell confluence or of some other effect imposed by a factor or factors in the medium, we grew two identical sets of normal keratinocytes for 3 days in KM, after which one set was fed with KM

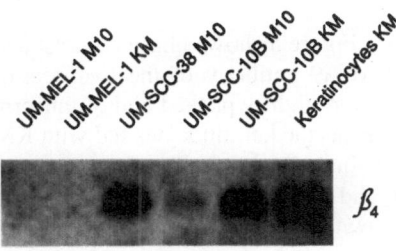

Figure 2. Northern analysis of β_4 mRNA from $\alpha^6\beta_4$ negative and positive cell lines grown in either M10 or KM.

73

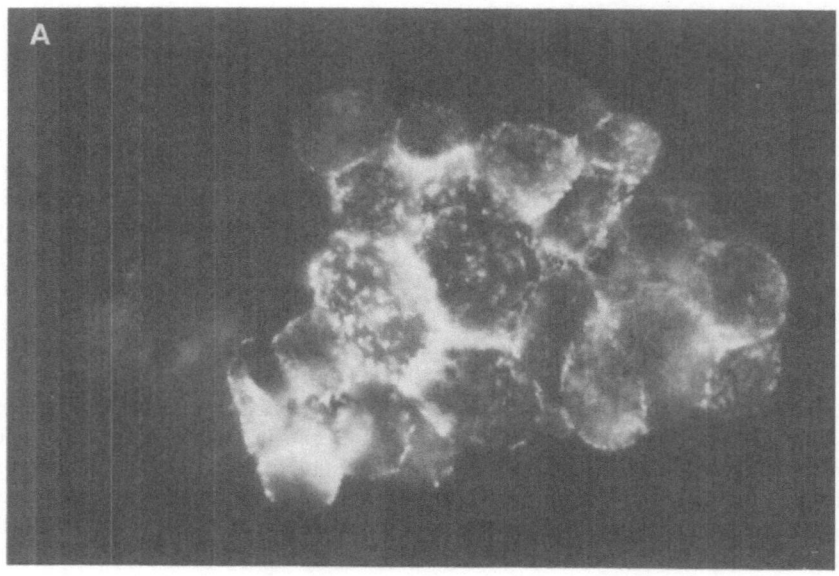

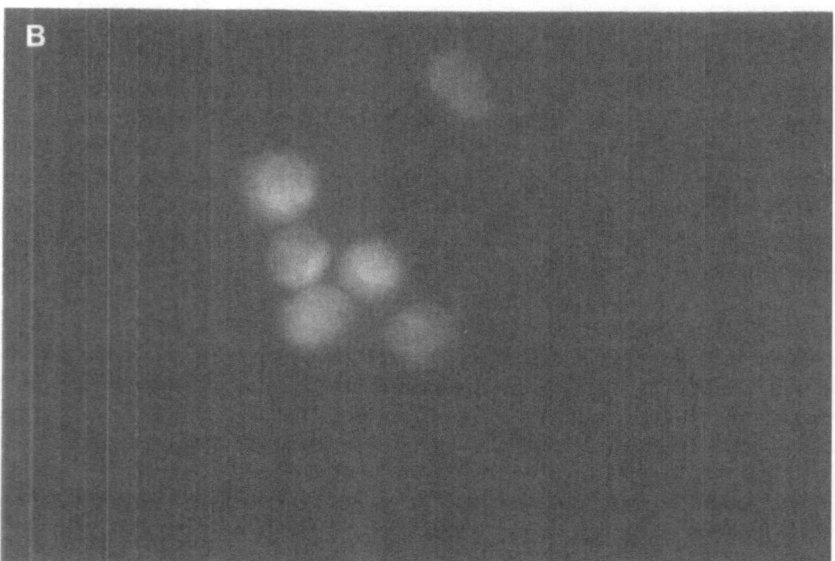

Figure 3. Indirect immunofluorescence staining of a suspension of UM-SCC-14C squamous carcinoma cells. (A) UM-SCC-14C cells stained with monoclonal antibody UM-A9; (B) UM-SCC-14C cells incubated with the isotype-matched control antibody 1B2B5 (100× objective).

for 6 additional days, and the other with M10 for 6 days. Figure 5 shows phase contrast and immunofluorescence photos after staining with the UM-A9 antibody of the two sets of cultures. The cells grown in KM became confluent and were tightly packed and of uniform size, with discreet spaces between cells (Figure 5A), whereas the keratinocytes fed with KM and M10 showed evidence of terminal differentiation, including a flattened appearance, increased cell–cell interactions, loss of nuclear detail, and pleomorphism for cell size and shape (Figure 5B). The immunofluorescence photos show that in the cultures fed with KM,

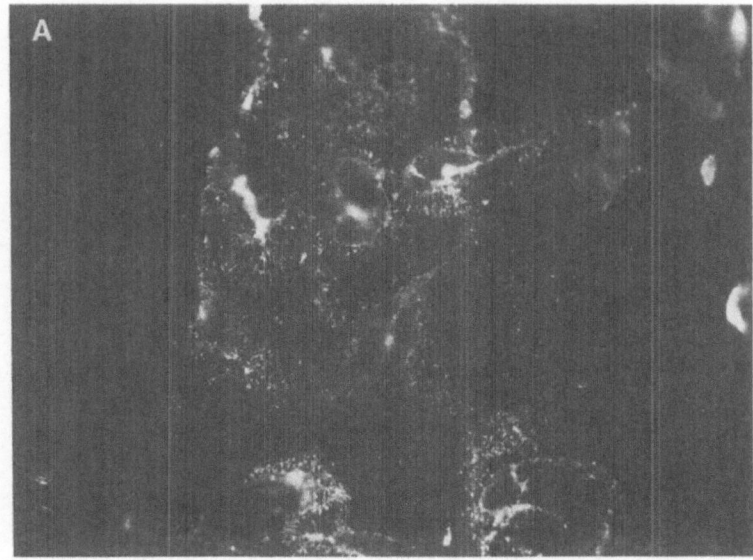

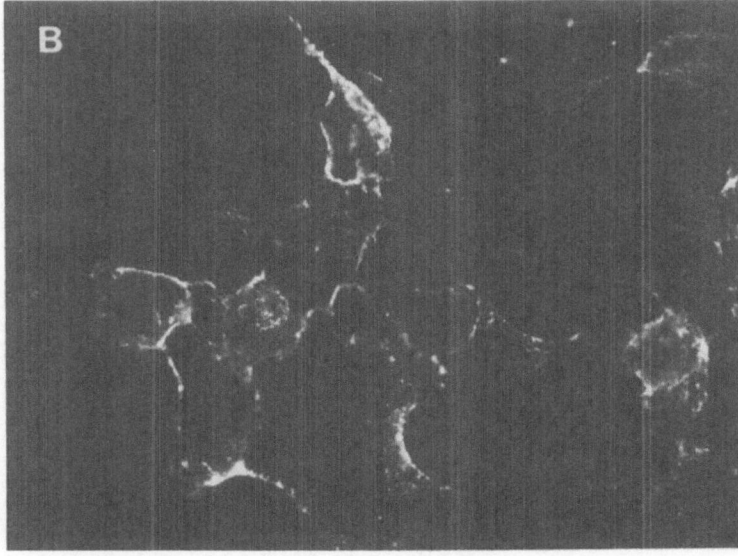

Figure 4. Indirect immunofluorescence photomicrographs of UM-SCC-14C cells grown on coverslips and stained with UM-A9 monoclonal antibody. (A) Cells grown in KM; (B) Cells grown in M10.

there was intense fluorescence in the spaces between cells (Figure 5C), whereas in the cultures fed with KM and M10, the intensity of fluorescence was reduced and could be detected only at the free boundaries of the cell colonies (Figure 5D).

DISCUSSION

Our previous results with tumor cell lines and tumor sections linked high-level expression of the A9/$\alpha^6\beta_4$ integrin to aggressive biologic behavior in SCCs (3–6). Based on those earlier findings, we had postulated that amplified expression of this integrin, at either the gene level or the transcriptional level, was responsible for the elevated level of antigen expression that we had documented in tumor cell lines and frozen sections of tumor tissues.

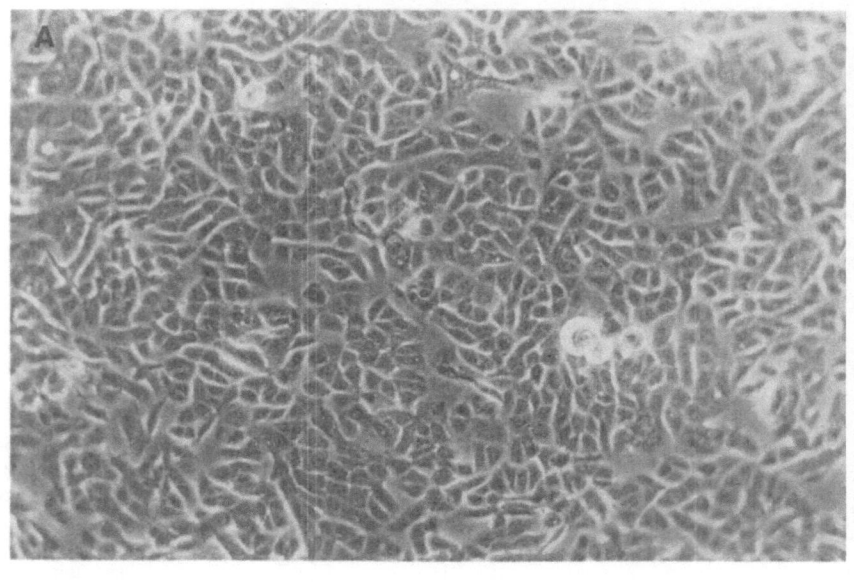

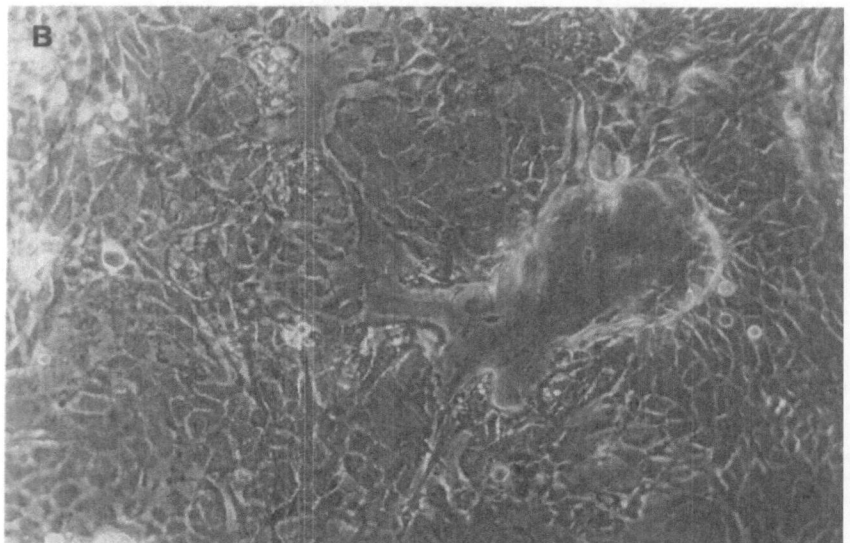

Figure 5. Phase contrast (A and B) and indirect immunofluorescence photomicrographs (C and D) of normal keratinocytes grown on coverslips for 9 days. Cells grown in KM for the entire period (A and C). Cells grown in KM for 3 days and then in M10 for 6 days (B and D).

The experiments described here, however, altered our perception of the relationship between high-level expression of $\alpha^6\beta_4$ and the behavior of tumors. When normal cells were grown under conditions that simulated the growth of undifferentiated tumor cells, high levels of expression resulted, both as message and as antigen. Nevertheless, the relationship between high A9/$\alpha^6\beta_4$ expression and tumorlike behavior still holds, since normal keratinoctyes have high A9/$\alpha^6\beta_4$ expression in conditions that foster rapid growth and migratory behavior, whereas the level of antigen expression falls when the cells are forced to differentiate.

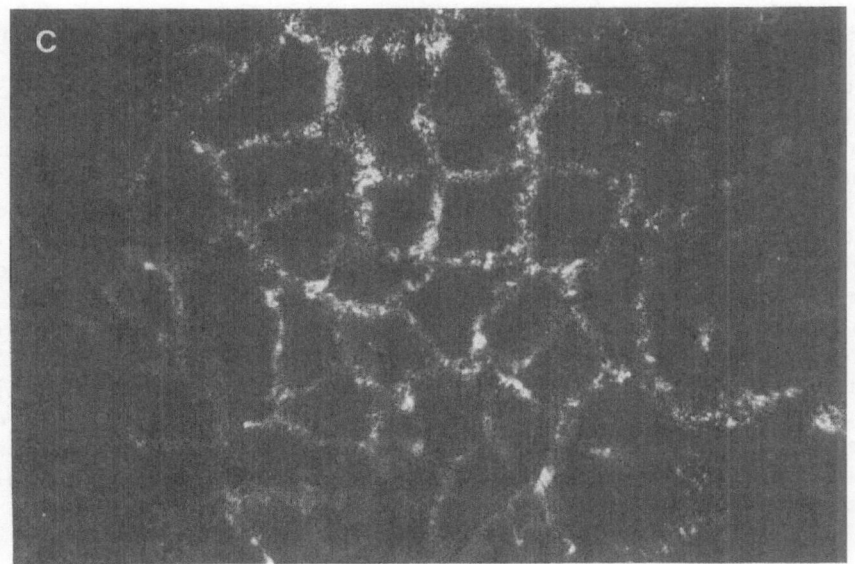

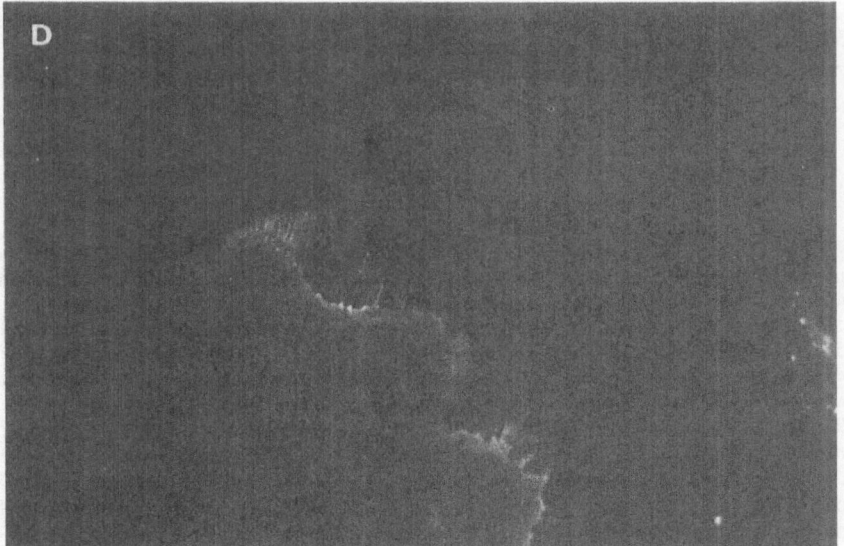

Our results are still very preliminary. A decrease in message in normal keratinocytes under conditions that favor differentiation has not been documented, nor has the time course necessary for expression to change been determined. Our results with α^6 message are still too preliminary to evaluate fully, but it seems clear that the β_4 message is not affected by EGF. It is not known why the mRNAs for α^6 and β_4 are lower in tumor cells grown in M10 than in the same types of cells grown in KM. These experiments suggest either that a component in KM other than EGF upregulates $\alpha^6\beta_4$ integrin message expression or that the M10 contains an inhibitory factor. The nature of the factor or factors that regulate $\alpha^6\beta_4$ expression has not been documented as of this writing. If expression of this integrin is linked to growth behavior, then identification of the signal that controls this gene will be very important in regulating the growth of squamous carcinomas. Future experiments will be directed at addressing these points and at determining whether regulators of cell differentiation, such as calcium and retinoic acid, can influence integrin expression.

Because it is very difficult to determine how in vitro manipulations affect tumor cell behavior in vivo, it is important to have a model that can be used both in vitro and in vivo in laboratory animals. The VX2 carcinoma is a long-established, transplantable squamous carcinoma of the rabbit (18) for which an in vitro analogue has been difficult to establish. There have been several previous reports (19–21) in the literature of other in vitro VX2 cell lines, but these cell lines are not readily available. A. Ptok and colleagues (unpublished data, 1991) recently established two in vitro cell lines from the VX2 carcinoma that have the capacity to induce, in nude mice, tumors that are identical to those caused by the parental rabbit VX2. These lines differ from each other in two ways. One line, UM-VX2-1, is adherent in culture and does not form tumors in rabbits unless the host is immunosuppressed with cyclosporin A. The other line, UM-VX2-2, is poorly adherent in culture and forms tumors in rabbits without immunosuppression. The failure of the latter line to adhere in vitro is suggestive of a defect or an alteration in expression of matrix receptors. We are just beginning to examine these cell lines to determine whether their altered behavior is accompanied by altered expression of the $\alpha^6\beta_4$ epithelial integrin.

ACKNOWLEDGMENTS

Supported by U.S. Public Health Service grant CA-35929, the University of Michigan Cancer Center (Ann Arbor, MI), the Biomedical Research Support grant, and the Office of the Vice President for Research at the University of Michigan.

The authors would like to acknowledge the help of Drs. Carolyn Damsky, Matt Harding, Martin Hemler, Mark Kaminski, Brian Nickoloff, and Arnoud Sonnenberg.

REFERENCES

1. Hong WK, Lippman SM, Itri LM, Karp DD, Lee JS, Byers RM, Schantz SP, Kramer AM, Lotan R, Peters LJ, Dimery IJ, Brown BW, Goepfert H. Prevention of second primary tumors with isotretinoin in squamous-cell carcinoma of the head and neck. N Engl J Med 323:795–801, 1990.
2. Lotan R. Effects of vitamin A and its analogs (retinoids) on normal and neoplastic cells. Biochim Biophys Acta 605:33–91, 1980.
3. Tong PS, Horowitz NN, Wheeler LA. Trans retinoic acid enhances the growth response of epidermal keratinocytes to epidermal growth factor and transforming growth factor beta. J Invest Dermatol 94:126–131, 1990.
4. Kimmel KA, Carey TE. Altered expression in squamous carcinoma cells of an orientation restricted epithelial antigen detected by monoclonal antibody A9. Cancer Res 46:3614–3623, 1986.
5. Wolf GT, Carey TE, Schmaltz SP, McClatchey KD, Poore J, Glaser L, Hayashida DJS, Hsu S. Altered antigen expression predicts outcome in squamous cell carcinoma of the head and neck. J Natl Cancer Inst 82:1566–1572, 1990.
6. Van Waes C, Kozarsky KF, Warren AB, Kidd L, Paugh D, Liebert M, Carey TE. The A9 antigen associated with aggressive human squamous carcinoma has structural and functional similarity to the newly defined integrin $\alpha^6\beta_4$. Cancer Res 51:2395–2402, 1991.
7. Hynes RO. Integrins: A family of cell surface receptors. Cell 48:549–554, 1987.
8. Boyce ST, Ham RG. Cultivation, frozen storage, and clonal growth of normal human epidermal keratinocytes in serum-free media. Journal of Tissue Culture Methods 9:83–93, 1985.
9. Sonnenberg A, Janssen H, Hogervorst F, Calafat J, Hilgers J. A complex of platelet glycoproteins Ic and IIa identified by a rat monoclonal antibody. J Biol Chem 262:10376–10383, 1987.
10. Chomczynski P, Sacchi N. Single-step method of RNA isolation by acid guanidinium thiocyanate-phenol-chloroform extraction. Anal Biochem 162:156–159, 1987.
11. Sambrook J, Fritsch EF, Maniatis T. Molecular Cloning: A Laboratory Manual, 2nd ed. New York: Cold Spring Harbor Laboratory Press, 1989.

12. Barker JNMN, Sarma V, Mitra RS, Dixit VM, Nickoloff BJ. Marked synergism between tumor necrosis factor-a and interferon g in regulation of keratinocyte-derived adhesion molecules and chemotactic factors. J Clin Invest 85:605–608, 1990.
13. Hemler ME, Crouse C, Sonnenberg A. Association of the VLA α^6 subunit with a novel protein: A possible alternative to the common VLA β_1 subunit on certain cell lines. J Biol Chem 264:6529–6539, 1989.
14. Hogervorst F, Kuikman I, von dem Borne AEG, Sonnenberg A. Cloning and sequence analysis of beta-4 cDNA: An integrin subunit that contains a unique 118 kd cytoplasmic domain. EMBO J 9:765–770, 1990.
15. Hogervorst F, Kuikman I, van Kessel AG, Sonnenberg A. Molecular cloning of the human α^6 integrin subunit and chromosomal location of the α^6 and β_4 genes. Eur J Biochem, in press.
16. Birnhorn HC, Doly J. A rapid alkaline extraction procedure for screening recombinant plasmid DNA. Nucleic Acids Res 7:1513, 1979.
17. Feinberg AP, Vogelstein B. A technique for radiolabelling DNA restriction endonuclease fragments to high specific activity. Anal Biochem 132:6–13, 1983.
18. Kidd JG, Rous P. A transplantable rabbit carcinoma originating in a virus-induced papilloma and containing the virus in masked or altered form. J Exp Med 71:813–838, 1940.
19. Easty DM, Easty GC. Establishment of an in vitro cell line from the rabbit VX2 carcinoma. Virchows Arch 39:333–337, 1982.
20. Georges E, Breitbund F, Jibard N, Orth G. Two Shope papillomavirus-associated VX2 carcinoma cell lines with different levels of keratinocyte differentiation and transplantability. J Virol 55:246–250, 1985.
21. Osato T, Ito Y. In vitro cultivation and immunofluorescent studies of transplantable carcinomas VX2 and VX7. J Exp Med 126:881–895, 1967.

Growth Factors and Other Targets for Rational Application as Intervention Agents

James L. Mulshine, Michael Birrer, Anthony M. Treston,
Frank Scott, Kathryn Quinn, Ingalill Avis, and Frank Cuttitta

Biomarkers and Prevention Research Branch
Education and Community Oncology Program
Division of Cancer Prevention and Cancer Control
National Cancer Institute
National Institutes of Health
Bethesda, Maryland

INTRODUCTION

Lung cancer is the leading cause of cancer deaths in the American society, with a mortality rate of close to 90% (1). The recalcitrance of lung cancer despite modern treatment approaches reflects the frequency of metastatic spread and the lack of effective systemic chemotherapeutic agents to eliminate disseminated cancer. Because of the lack of progress in treating metastatic lung cancer, new strategies for lung cancer control (prevention, early detection, and intervention) are being studied. Primary prevention efforts, such as the California state government's large cigarette sales tax mandated by Proposition 99, are beginning to show remarkable results in reducing cigarette consumption (2). Efforts to improve the early detection of lung cancer are also beginning to show signs of promise (3–5). Complementing these are positive developments in the area of intervention therapy for very early lung cancer.

Two recent trials suggest that lung cancer may be amenable in its early phases to intervention approaches that involve vitamin A derivatives. The first trial involved a group of 100 patients with head and neck cancer who were randomly assigned to receive either 100 mg/ m^2 of 13-*cis*–retinoic acid or a placebo daily for 1 year after a definitive standard treatment for their initial head and neck cancer (6). Head and neck cancer patients have a high rate of developing second primary cancers, especially in the lungs and other upper aerodigestive sites. After 3 years, the group who received 13-*cis*–retinoic acid had developed significantly fewer new primary cancers than had the placebo group (two new primary cancers, including no lung cancers, compared with a total of 15 cancers in the placebo-treated group, including three new lung cancers).

In the preliminary analysis of a trial of patients with Stage I resected non–small cell lung cancer, a group of patients randomly selected to receive retinol palmitate had a significant prolongation of their relapse-free survival compared with untreated control patients (7). Although it is too early to ascribe definite benefit to chemointervention with retinoids for populations at high risk for developing lung cancer, the results of these trials suggest that this clinically silent phase of lung cancer may be amenable to control, as has been predicted (8).

The Biology and Prevention of Aerodigestive Tract Cancers
Edited by G.R.Newell and W.K. Hong, Plenum Press, New York, 1992

81

During the clinically silent phase of lung carcinogenesis, when the malignant clone is expanding on the respiratory mucosa, there is still no consistent way to detect the nascent malignancy. Specific knowledge of the biology of lung cancer during this phase is very limited, as there are no diagnostic tools capable of identifying the disease at this stage. The need for developing effective early-detection tools for lung cancer is compelling since tools that can detect early lung cancer may have dual application, either as early detection markers or as surrogate marker to guage the success of rational intervention efforts. Research efforts into early detection and intervention have considerable potential for cross-fertilization.

Further clinical evaluation of retinoid-based interventions with early lung cancer will also need to address a wide range of issues, including the optimal-range dose and the formulation and duration of therapy. As these basic issues are resolved, more benefits of retinoid-based intervention for early lung cancer may become evident.

LUNG GROWTH FACTORS AS RATIONAL INTERVENTION TARGETS

The preliminary success with retinoids has redirected attention to intervention research as a promising area for improving lung cancer control. Lung cancer growth factors are attractive targets for intervention. Lung cancer cells produce and respond to a number of growth factors, including gastrin-releasing peptide (GRP) (9), insulin-like growth factor I (IGF-I) (10), a transferrin-like molecule (11-13), and epidermal growth factor (EGF) (14,15). These growth factors may play a role in a variety of normal processes underlying lung development, repair of injury, and lung carcinogenesis.

Much is known about GRP, which may provide a model for lung cancer intervention research. Evidence is mounting that GRP plays a significant role in fetal lung growth and maturation (16,17). Investigators at the University of Colorado have shown that a GRP-like substance is elevated in the bronchial lavage of healthy smokers compared to nonsmokers (18). These data suggest that growth factors may be cancer promotion factors and may play a major role in cancer progression.

A clinical trial is under way using a neutralizing antibody to GRP to evaluate the clinical benefit of a sustained immunologic blockade of GRP effect (19). The Phase I experience in a population of patients with relapsed lung cancer has demonstrated that repeated doses of a neutralizing anti-GRP monoclonal antibody (up to 12 doses over 28 days) have been well tolerated (no obvious clinical toxicity); unfortunately, no antitumor effects were noted (20). However, the prospects for meaningful clinical intervention by an agent should not be discounted simply because of its lack of effectiveness as an agent in treating advanced metastatic disease. This ineffectiveness was also the preliminary experience with retinoids; Lippman and co-workers had found that advanced head and neck cancers were not significantly responsive to treatment with 13-*cis*–retinoic acid alone (21). In theory at least, early cancers are potentially more amenable to pharmacologic inhibition because of the combined effect of a smaller tumor burden and the more restricted genetic diversity of early cancers.

A number of reports describe antibodies that neutralize the growth effects of other lung cancer growth factors (10,12–15). Current knowledge may not be sufficient to answer definitively which growth factor is the most important in mediating tumor progression. However, since the previously cited work of the Colorado group suggests that growth factor quantitation from normal lung secretions is feasible (18), systematic evaluation of the quality and quantity of growth factor expression in the airways of individuals at high risk for cancer could provide important data on growth factor dynamics, which in turn could influence the development of growth factor-based intervention approaches.

Because lung cancer appears as a number of different histologies that may arise from different types of tissues in response to different types of carcinogen exposure, it is likely that more than one growth factor may be functioning as a tumor promoter (22,23). If more than one growth factor antagonist is used in combination to neutralize multiple progression factors, the treatment will have the potential for greater host toxicity. Therefore, careful preclinical studies in relevant model systems will need to be performed to clarify potential risks of combined anti-growth factor intervention. Moreover, because all of the previously mentioned growth factors play a role in normal biologic functions, the possibility of unintended consequences of growth factor-based interventions must be carefully evaluated in the Phase I and II evaluations. This type of application demands a very precise understanding of normal tissue and tumor biology to define the optimal biologic dose.

Because the anticipated target for intervention therapy in lung cancer is the respiratory epithelium, the possibility exists to deliver intervention agents via the airway instead of the systemic circulatory system. The pharmacologic benefits of such direct intra-airway delivery in terms of specific targeting efficiency could be considerable.

CONSIDERATION IN GROWTH FACTOR MODULATION AS A RATIONAL INTERVENTION APPROACH

In interventions using anti-growth factors, a number of theoretical concerns are relevant. One important concern is targeting a normal growth factor to inhibit tumor promotion. This precedent will soon be addressed in a major anti-estrogen–based intervention trial of breast cancer (24,25). Estrogen is considered a key promotional agent in the development of breast cancer (24,25). Endogenous estrogenic activity can be produced in a variety of normal sites, including the adrenals, ovaries, and peripheral adipose tissues. The peripheral production of estrogenlike compounds is thought to greatly influence the increased incidence of breast cancer in countries where the diet is high in fat. The high levels of unopposed exposure of breast ductal epithelium to estrogen is likely to be greatest in developed countries like the United States, where food is easy to get, the common life-style is sedentary, and females experience early menses, late initial childbearing, and late menopause.

The impetus for the tamoxifen intervention trial arises from a retrospective analysis of adjuvant breast cancer trials, groups of women who received chronic adjuvant anti-estrogen tamoxifen therapy for a primary ipsilateral breast cancer were found to have a 40% reduction in the incidence of second primary breast cancers in the contralateral breast (25). This reduction was reproducible in large groups of women. Two pilot trials, one in Scotland and one in the United States, have tested the initial feasibility of an anti-estrogen–based intervention approach (26,27). Of major concern was whether the biochemical neutralization of estrogen would have an unintended adverse effect on bone density and cardiovascular disease (24,25). The preliminary results of the anti-estrogen therapy appeared to show dissimilar effects, with the desired antagonism in tumor tissue but, surprisingly, an estrogenlike effect in bone and cardiovascular tissue. This outcome implies that the biology of the estrogen receptors of normal and malignant tissue is different; however, further verification is needed.

Also not established in the various pilot tamoxifen intervention studies was the optimal level of anti-estrogen effect for the mediation of an anti-breast cancer effect, whether the estrogen effects should be blocked completely, how long they should be blocked, and when the block should be started are questions that should be considered in the context of an ethnically mixed and genetically diverse patient population. Also, because breast cancer may not be a single disease, variable degrees of estrogen dependence would be expected. As with lung cancer, a number of other growth factors may be relevant to breast cancer promotion. Because the extent and timing of the growth factor interactions may be difficult to identify precisely, very careful analysis of these complex interactions is required. Thus, for breast cancer and lung cancer, the development of analytical tools to evaluate growth factor dynamics in individual patients and refine anti-growth factor interventions is an exciting area for investigative efforts.

The successful development of anti-growth factor interventions implies a long-term commitment to evaluate systematically the biology of these dynamics. Pharmacologic tools that will serially measure the pharmacokinetics and pharmacodynamics of the intervention agent in study populations must be developed. Reliable methods of pharmacologic monitoring of the intervention agent must also be developed to address the degree of subject compliance and the adequacy of individual dosing.

Developing intervention strategies for breast cancer and lung cancer will involve many parallel features, including, for example, whether a threshold level of a particular promotion factor is critical to tumor progression. Again, when the epidemiologic data for breast cancer is considered, a major difference variation in breast cancer rates can be seen among certain populations. These data suggest that exposure to low levels of estrogen is not always a significant cancer promotion factor. The ultimate goal of anti-estrogen cancer intervention may be to reduce the levels of estrogen, at least during critical developmental periods, to the mean exposure level of that seen in populations with lower breast cancer incidence. By maintaining some level of estrogen, women may be spared the morbidity related to the premature menopause that results from estrogen loss.

Defining the levels of tumor promotion factors associated with increased frequency of carcinogenesis provides a basis for rational intervention approaches. Formulating such interventions requires the close cooperation of investigators in the applied and basic sciences. Much of the initial work related to interventions for breast cancer will contribute to strategies also appropriate for other epithelial cancers, including lung cancer.

To make clinical research into effective tumor intervention approaches more economical, markers must be developed that will more readily identify the population at risk of developing cancer. The development of new prevention-orientated clinical trial structures is essential and will entail methodologies that depart from typical Phase I, II, and III cancer trials.

The target population for intervention trials will consist of healthy people, who may be less compliant than patients with advanced cancer. Subject awareness programs that are sensitive to culture and the community must be developed to encourage fuller understanding, participation, and compliance with the particular intervention approach. Both the "hard" science issues of tumor biology and rational biochemical interventions and the "soft" social science issues regarding study participation and compliance must be carefully reconciled to stimulate the rate of research in this new direction.

RELATIONSHIP OF INTERVENTION APPROACHES TO EARLY LUNG CANCER DETECTION

The identification of lung tumors confined solely to the bronchial epithelium would imply either that physicians would be able to detect lung cancer at a much earlier phase than is currently possible or that as a function of the clinical trial design, a population at high risk for lung cancer would be defined to include a certain number of people who would probably have undiagnosed, very early lung cancer. In the latter situation, a clinical trial end point could be a significant reduction in the development of new lung cancers among people in this high-risk population, compared with a control population. An example of this approach is the previously discussed trial investigating the use of 13-*cis*–retinoic acid in patients with head and neck cancer (6).

We have reported an approach to early lung cancer detection involving sputum immunostaining with tumor-associated monoclonal antibodies, a procedure that can identify lung cancer cases with 90% accuracy approximately 2 years prior to routine clinical detection (3). The details of this approach have been previously reviewed (3,4). There are two important findings from this research. The first is that the earliest detection of lung cancer usually occurs by monitoring the specific compartment where the lung cancer arises: the bronchial epithelium. Sputum from an individual with an early cancer may contain a number of cells that reveal the presence of the malignancy. Based on a prospective analysis of conventional sputum cytology as an early-detection tool for lung cancer, detection with this method can be done in only about 10% of patients. Our research has shown that in contrast to this ineffective approach, sputum immunocytochemistry is successful as an early-detection tool. This latter assay utilizes monoclonal antibodies that recognize particular cellular targets overexpressed by cells involved in early lung carcinogenesis. These cells are shed from the bronchial epithelium and recovered in the sputum. A second finding is that conceivably, a number of quantitative or qualitative changes in dysplastic bronchial epithelial cells may indicate that cellular transformation has occurred. It is also possible that a panel of markers, including more than just two antibody markers used for identifying individuals with early lung cancer, would be more accurate than any individual marker (3). In addition to analyzing for growth factors or cell surface changes, using specific genetic targets could further enhance the effectiveness of this approach.

MOLECULAR CHANGES DURING LUNG CARCINOGENESIS

Recent discoveries in the genetics of lung cancer have identified key target genes that undergo genetic mutations during tumor development (28,29). These genetic events clearly underlie the pathologic changes characteristic of the multistage process of human epithelial carcinogenesis (30). These genes include many nuclear and cytoplasmic oncogenes and growth factors and their receptors. Although great progress has been made in identifying and characterizing these genes, their precise clinical relevance and the chronological occurrence of mutations in them during lung carcinogenesis remain unknown. One of the major challenges for future research will be to determine which one or ones of these mutations are early activation events in lung cancer and, as such, whether they can be useful markers for early disease.

Of the genes identified so far, the most promising include the *ras* gene family, *Her-2/neu*, and *p53* (29,31). The Kirsten *ras* gene is mutated in approximately 30% of all adenocarcinomas of the lung (32). These point mutations result in activation of the gene, the presence of which has been shown to correlate with a poor clinical prognosis (33). The techniques of modern molecular biology allow the detection, in small amounts of tissue, of these single codon mutations, which activate this gene. The polymerase chain reaction (PCR) provides amplification of the Kirsten *ras* gene potentially from as little tissue as a single cell (34). Analysis of these amplified sequences can be undertaken by several techniques: 1) differential hybridization to a radiolabeled fragment of mutated oligonucleotides (35), 2) identification of new restriction sites created by the activating mutations (36), 3) single-strand conformational polymorphism (SSCP) (37), and 4) direct nucleic acid sequencing. Using these approaches, scientists may be able to detect the presence of activated *ras* genes in relatively small tissue samples, such as biopsies of premalignant dysplastic bronchial tissue, sputum samples, or both. Although activated *ras* genes are found in only 15% of all lung cancers, because they are limited primarily to adenocarcinomas, they may provide additional sensitivity and specificity to other screening techniques that do not work well in this subset of lung tumors.

Mutations in the nuclear proto-oncogene *p53* have been frequently detected in a wide range of tumors, including those in the colon, breast, and lung (38). Whether these mutations occur as early or late events during tumor development remains unknown. Examination of dysplastic and metaplastic bronchial epithelium for this particular genetic lesion will be critical in determining the potential role of *p53* as an activation event. This gene and its mutations can be analyzed in a fashion similar to that just described. The technology exists for PCR amplification of the *p53* gene, which in turn can be analyzed for point mutations or small deletions. This analysis can be accomplished by SSCP, RNAase protection, or direct nucleic acid sequencing (39,40). These approaches can detect the majority of mutations in this gene, although inactivating mutations outside the coding region and in the promoter would be missed. A complementary approach that examines only the protein end product is immunohistochemical staining using antibodies directed at the wild type and mutant forms of the gene. Although this technique also has limitations, it can be applied to small numbers of cells (even single cells) and can possibly detect increased levels of a mutated p53 protein resulting from any of the above events.

Finally, the *Her-2/neu* oncogene has been detected as amplified and overexpressed in several epithelial cancers, including a subset of lung cancer tumors. In better characterized tumors, such as breast cancer, overexpression of this oncogene correlates with a more aggressive phenotype and a poorer prognosis for the patient. Since well-characterized antisera already exist, this would clearly be another molecular change that could be used to detect early malignant changes in epithelial cells of the lung.

Of course, there are many other potential genetic targets, such as *myc, ras, jun, fos*, and *Rb*, that may ultimately serve as markers for the multistage process of epithelial carcinogenesis (29,31). Unfortunately, at present these genes are found less consistently involved in lung cancer and are also less amenable than those listed above to systematic evaluation on small amounts of tissue. However, as technology expands and the early events in lung cancer become more clearly understood, many of these markers may be routinely used to screen patients for early lung cancer.

In summary, although man's understanding of the genetic events that occur in early lung carcinogenesis is still limited, the probability of molecular, genetic-based early detection has become a reality. Many suspected genetic lesions can be elucidated by applying known techniques to volumes of tissues generally available in common clinical practices. The potential application of prevention-based approaches to lung cancer control based on the rational application of tumor biology provides exciting research opportunities, with the long-term promise of significant clinical benefit.

ACKNOWLEDGMENT

Portions of this work were supported by a generous grant from the Leila Y. and Harold G. Mathers Foundation.

REFERENCES

1. Boring CC, Squires TS, Tong T. Cancer statistics. CA: A Cancer Journal for Clinicians 41:19–36, 1991.
2. Bal DG, Kizer KW, Felton PG, Mozar HN, Niemeyer D. Reducing tobacco consumption in California: Development of a statewide anti-tobacco use campaign. JAMA 264:1570–1574, 1990.
3. Tockman MS, Levin ML, Frost JK, Ball WC Jr. Screening and detection of lung cancer. In Aisner J (ed): Lung Cancer. New York: Churchill Livingstone, 1985, pp. 25-48.
4. Mulshine JL, Tockman MS, Smart CR. Considerations in the development of lung cancer screening tools. J Natl Cancer Inst 81:900–906, 1989.
5. Mulshine JL, Magnani JL, Linnoila RI. Applications of monoclonal antibodies in the treatment of solid tumors. In DeVita V, Rosenberg S, Hellman S (eds): Biologic Therapy of Cancer. Philadelphia: JB Lippincott, 1991, pp. 563-582.
6. Hong WK, Lippman SM, Itri LM, Karp D, Lee J, Byers R, Schantes S, Kramer A, Lotan R, Peters L, Dimery I, Brown B, Goepfert H. Prevention of second primary tumors in squamous cell carcinoma of the head and neck with 13-*cis*-retinoic acid. N Engl J Med 323:795–801, 1990.
7. Lippman SM, Hittelman WN, Lotan R, Pastorino U, Hong WK. Recent advances in cancer chemoprevention. Cancer Cells 3:59–65, 1991.
8. Sporn MB, Roberts AB. Role of retinoids in differentiation and carcinogenesis. Cancer Res 43:3034-3039, 1983.
9. Cuttitta F, Carney DN, Mulshine JL, Moody TW, Fedorko J, Fischler A, Minna JD. Bombesin-like peptides can

function as autocrine growth factors in human small-cell lung cancer. Nature 316:823–826, 1985.

10. Nakanishi Y, Mulshine JL, Kasprzyk P, Natale RB, Maneckijee R, Avis I, Treston AM, Gazdar A, Minna J, Cuttitta F. Small cell lung cancer cells autostimulate their growth via an insulin-like growth factor-I activity: Evaluation of 4 cell lines. J Clin Invest 82:354–359, 1988.

11. Vostrejs M, Moran PL, Seligman PA. Transferrin synthesis by small cell lung cancer cells acts as an autocrine regulator of cellular proliferation. J Clin Invest 82:331–339, 1988.

12. Nakanishi Y, Cuttitta F, Kasprzyk PG, Avis I, Steinberg SM, Gazdar AF, Mulshine JL. Growth factor effects on small cell lung cancer using a colorimetric assay: Can a transferrin-like factor mediate autocrine growth? Experimental Cell Biology 56:74–85, 1988.

13. Mulshine JL, Natale RB, Avis I, Treston A, Kasprzyk P, Nakanishi Y, Sausville E, Trepel JB, Cuttitta F. Autocrine growth factors and lung cancer. In Hansen H (ed): Basic and Clinical Concepts of Lung Cancer. Boston: Kluwer Academic Publisher, 1989, pp. 107-122.

14. Divgi DR, Welt SK, Yeh SDJ, Real F, Gralla R, Kris M, Masui H, Mendelsohn J. Phase I and imaging trial with radiolabeled anti EGF receptor mons 225 (mAB) in squamous. Proceedings of the American Society of Clinical Oncology 88:183, 1989.

15. Lee M, Draoui M, Zia F, Gazdar A, Oie H, Bepler G, Bellot F, Tarr C, Kris R, Moody TM. Epidermal growth factor receptor monoclonal antibodies inhibit the growth of lung cancer cell lines. J Natl Cancer Inst (in press).

16. Sunday ME, Hua J, Dai HB, Nusrat A, Torday JS. Bombesin increases fetal lung growth and maturation in utero and in organ culture. Am J Respir Cell Mol Biol 3:199–205, 1990.

17. Wharton J, Polak JM, Bloom SR, Ghatei MA, Solcia E, Brown MR, Pearse AGE. Bombesin-like immunoreactivity in the lung. Nature 273:769–770, 1978.

18. Aguayo SM, Kane M, Schwarz MI, Graver L, Miller YE. Increased levels of bombesin-like peptides in the lower respiratory tracts of asymptomatic cigarette smokers. J Clin Invest 84:1105–1113, 1989.

19. Mulshine JL, Avis I, Treston AM, Kasprzyk P, Mobley C, Carrasquillo JA, Larson SM, Nakanishi Y, Merchant B, Minna JD, Cuttitta F. Clinical use of monoclonal antibody to bombesin-like peptide in patients with lung cancer. Ann N Y Acad Sci 547:360–372, 1989.

20. Mulshine JL, Avis I, Carrasquillo JA, Merchant B, Boland C, Perentesis P, Reynolds J, Larson S, Treston A, Scott F, Kasprzyk P, Johnson B, Ihde D, Gazdar A, Cuttitta F, Minna J. Phase I study of an anti-gastrin releasing peptide (GRP) monoclonal antibody in patients with lung cancer. Proceedings of the American Society of Clinical Oncology 9:230, 1990.

21. Lippman SM, Kessler JF, Al-Sarraf M, Alberts DS, Merchant B, Boland C, Perentesis P, Reynolds J, Larson S, Treston A, Scott F, Kasprzyk P, Johnson B, Ihde D, Gazdar A, Cuttitta F, Minna J. Treatment of advanced squamous cell carcinoma of the head and neck with isotretinoin: A phase II randomized trial. Invest New Drugs 6:51–56, 1988.

22. Gazdar AF, McDowell EM. Pathobiology of lung cancer. In Rosen S, Mulshine J, Cuttitta F, Abrams P (eds): Biology of Lung Cancer. New York: Marcel Dekker, 1988, pp. 1-34.

23. Mulshine JL, Linnoila RI, Magnani J. Application of monoclonal antibodies in the management of lung cancer patients. In Pass H (ed): Chest Surgery Clinics of North America 1:1–37, 1991.

24. Love RR. Commentary: Prospects for antiestrogen chemoprevention of breast cancer. J Natl Cancer Inst 82:18–21, 1990.

25. Jordan VC. Long-term tamoxifen: Balancing benefits and risks. Contemporary Oncology, March/April:26–33, 1991.

26. Fornander T, Rutqvist LE, Cedermark B, Mattsson A, Skoog L, Theve T, Askergren J, Rutqvist L, Glas U, Silfversward C, Somell A, Wilking N, Hjalmar M. Adjuvant tamoxifen in early breast cancer: Occurrence of new primary cancers. Lancet 1:117-120, 1989.

27. Fisher B, Costantino J, Redmond C, Poisson R, Bowman D, Couture J, Dimitrov N, Wolmark N, Wickerham D, Fisher E, Margolese R, Robidoux A, Shibata H, Terz J, Paterson A, Feldman M, Farra W, Evans J, Lickley H, Ketner M. A randomized clinical trial evaluating tamoxifen in the treatment of patients with node-negative breast cancer who have estrogen-receptor-positive tumors. N Engl J Med 320:479-484, 1989.

28. Whang-Peng J, Knutsen T, Gazdar A, Steinberg SM, Oie H, Linnoila I, Mulshine JL, Nau M, Minna JD. Nonrandom structural and numerical changes in non-small-cell lung cancer. Genes, Chromosomes & Cancer 8:39–41, 1991.

29. Birrer MJ, Minna JD. Molecular genetics of lung cancer. Semin Oncol 15:226–235, 1988.

30. Weinberg RA. Oncogenes and multistep carcinogenesis. In Weinberg RA (ed): Oncogenes and the Molecular Origins of Cancer, vol 18. New York: Cold Spring Harbor Laboratory, 1989, pp. 307-327.

31. Birrer MJ, Minna JD. Genetic changes in the pathogenesis of lung cancer. Annu Rev Med 40:305–317, 1989.

32. Rodenhuis S, Van der Wetering M, Mooi S, Evers SG, Van Zandwijk N, Bos J. Mutational activation of the K-ras oncogene: A possible pathogenetic factor in adenocarcinoma of the lung. N Engl J Med 317:929–935, 1987.

33. Slebos RJC, Kibbelaar RE, Dalesio O, Kooistra A, Stam J, Meijer C, Wagenaar S, Vanderschueren R, Van Zandwijk N, Mooi WJ, Bos J, Rodenhuis S. K-ras oncogene activation as a prognostic marker in adenocarcinoma of the lung. N Engl J Med 323:561–565, 1990.

34. Saiki RK, Scharf S, Faloona F, Mullis KB, Horn GT, Erlich HA, Arnheim N. Enzymatic amplification of β-globin genomic sequences and restriction site analysis for diagnosis of sickle cell anemia. Science 230:1350–1354, 1985.

35. Verlaan de Vries M, Bogaard ME, Van den Elsts H, Van Boom JH, Van der Eb AJ, Bos JL. A dot-blot screening procedure for mutated *ras* oncogenes using synthetic oligodeoxynucleotides. Gene 50:313–320, 1986.

36. Jiang W, Kahn SM, Guillem JG, Lu S, Weinstein IB. Rapid detection of *ras* oncogenes in human tumors: Application to colon, esophageal, and gastric cancers. Oncogene 4:923–928, 1989.

37. Suzuki Y, Orita M, Shiraishi M, Hayashi K, Sekiya T. Detection of *ras* gene mutations in human lung cancers by single-strand conformation polymorphism analysis of polymerase chain reacting products. Oncogene 5:1037–1043, 1990.

38. Baker S, Fearon E, Nigro J, Hamilton S, Preisinger A, Jessup J, Van Tuinen P, Ledbetter D, Nakamura Y, White R, Vogelstein B, Baker D. Chromosome 17 deletions of *p53* gene mutations in colorectal carcinomas. Science 244:217–221, 1989.

39. Takahashi T, Nau M, Chiba I, Buchhagen D, Minna J. *p53*: A frequent target for genetic abnormalities in lung cancer. Science 246:491–494, 1989.

40. Chiba I, Takahashi T, Nau MM, D'Amico D, Curiel DT, Mitsudomi T, Buchhagen DL, Carbone D, Piantadosi S, Koga H, Reissman PT, Slamon DJ, Homes EC, Minna JD. Mutations in the *p53* gene are frequent in primary resected non-small cell lung cancer. Oncogene 5:1603–1610, 1990.

Hyperplasia and Squamous Metaplasia in the Tracheobronchial Epithelium: Alterations in the Balance of Growth and Differentiation Factors

Anton M. Jetten, Thomas M. Vollberg, and Clara Nervi

Cell Biology Section
Laboratory of Pulmonary Pathobiology
National Institute of Environmental Health Sciences
Research Triangle Park, North Carolina

The tracheobronchial epithelium is a continuously self-renewing columnar, pseudo-stratified epithelium. During regular turnover of this epithelium, terminally differentiated cells are replaced through the proliferation and differentiation of progenitor cells (1). Under normal conditions, the rate of renewal is relatively slow. To maintain the normal structure of the epithelium, the rates of proliferation and differentiation and cell loss must be equal. Various growth and differentiation factors, including several polypeptide growth factors, cytokines, and retinoids, cooperate to maintain this balance. During development, a different balance of growth and differentiation factors is required to sustain the rapid growth of the tissue. Changes in the synthesis or activation of these factors are one likely cause of increased proliferation under certain pathologic conditions, including hyperplasia, squamous metaplasia, and neoplasia. The tracheobronchial epithelium contains several cell types (basal, neuroendocrine, and mucous cells) that are able to undergo mitosis. Increased proliferation of these cell types may lead to either basal cell, mucous cell, or neuroendocrine cell hyperplasia. It is likely that the hyperproliferation of these three cell types is regulated differently and controlled by different factors. In this chapter, we will focus on studies designed to understand basal cell hyperplasia.

HYPERPLASIA

Since the tracheobronchial epithelium renews itself rather slowly, many progenitor cells can remain in the quiescent (G_0) phase of the cell cycle (Figure 1). During hyperplasia, these cells can be recruited to reenter the cell cycle. This process is also initiated when tracheobronchial epithelial cells are placed in culture in the presence of growth-enhancing factors (1–3). A number of such growth factors that could play a role in hyperplasia have been identified. Epidermal growth factor (EGF), transforming growth factor-α (TGF-α), insulin, insulinlike growth factor I (IGFI), and keratinocyte growth factor (KGF) have been reported to stimulate the growth of tracheobronchial epithelial cells. These factors can act on such cells by autocrine or paracrine mechanisms. For instance, the presence of EGF receptors and the ability to synthesize and release TGF-α may constitute, in tracheobronchial epithelial cells, two seg-

The Biology and Prevention of Aerodigestive Tract Cancers
Edited by G.R.Newell and W.K. Hong, Plenum Press, New York, 1992

89

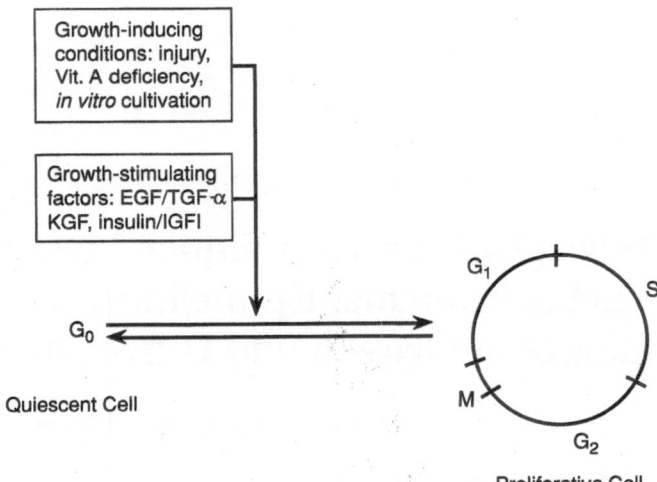

Figure 1. Induction of hyperproliferation in tracheobronchial epithelial cells. Many progenitor cells are in the quiescent (G_0) phase of the cell cycle. Injury, vitamin A deficiency, and in vitro cultivation cause hyperproliferation. This may be due to increased synthesis or activation of positive growth factors (e.g., EGF/TGF-α, insulin/IGFI, or KGF) that induce quiescent cells to reenter the cell cycle.

ments of an autocrine loop. In addition, lung fibroblasts and macrophages are able to synthesize TGF-α that could induce proliferation of tracheobronchial epithelial cells by a paracrine mechanism. In the normal tracheobronchial epithelium, the levels of active TGF-α may be relatively low, and increased synthesis or activation of TGF-α may result in a stimulation of proliferation of tracheobronchial epithelial cells and result in hyperplasia. A role for EGF/TGF-α in hyperplasia is supported by the findings of Stahlman et al. (4), showing that increased levels of EGF can cause hyperplasia in the tracheobronchial epithelium of fetal lambs.

In culture, optimal growth of tracheobronchial epithelial cells is dependent on the presence of insulin or IGFI. IGFI is 50–100 times more potent than insulin in stimulating the growth of such cells, suggesting that these growth factors act via the type I IGF receptor. This is confirmed by studies showing that tracheobronchial epithelial cells contain type I IGF receptors (2). Tracheobronchial epithelial cells do not produce IGFI; however, lung fibroblasts and alveolar macrophages have been shown to secrete IGFI, which may regulate growth and differentiation of tracheobronchial epithelial cells in a paracrine manner. KGF, a member of the fibroblast growth factor family (1,5), is synthesized by lung fibroblasts and has been shown to enhance the growth of cultured tracheobronchial epithelial cells. The observations above suggest that growth factors produced by several cell types may participate in the process that induces hyperplasia in the airways.

Neoplastic cells have been reported to exhibit an altered regulation of cell growth. In these cells, the regulated control of proliferation can be disrupted at several levels. In some cases, the disruption can result from the constitutive production of one or more positive growth factors. Increased synthesis of TGF-α and IGFI has been reported in several lung carcinoma cell lines (6). Other defects implicate growth factor receptors and other genes that play a role in the signal transduction pathway of growth factors (7).

IRREVERSIBLE GROWTH ARREST

In the tracheobronchial epithelium, basal cell hyperplasia is not an uncontrolled process. In vivo, when cells stratify, the upper layers undergo a pathway of squamous differentiation (8). Irreversible growth arrest is the first step in this terminal differentiation process and appears to be a prerequisite for the expression of the squamous-differentiated phenotype. In vitro, irreversible growth arrest can be induced by the addition of phorbol esters or interferon-γ and occurs when cultures reach confluence (8–10). It is likely that some of the changes in gene expression that accompany irreversible and reversible growth arrest are identical. Although these have not yet been identified, certain changes in gene expression are probably unique to the induction of irreversible growth arrest. Defects in such genes may reduce the probability of the cells to become irreversibly growth arrested and to undergo terminal differentiation, thereby contributing to the neoplastic nature of the affected cell.

EXPRESSION OF THE SQUAMOUS-DIFFERENTIATED PHENOTYPE

After the cells are committed to irreversible growth arrest, they begin to express the squamous-differentiated phenotype (1,8). Many biochemical and molecular markers have been identified that characterize this differentiated phenotype. An increase in cholesterol sulfate and transglutaminase type I are among the earlier markers of differentiation (9–11). The increase in cholesterol sulfate has been reported to be related to an increase in cholesterol sulfotransferase activity (12). Recently, we have isolated a cDNA clone encoding the transglutaminase type I mRNA and demonstrated that the increase in transglutaminase activity is related to an increase in both corresponding protein and mRNA levels (9,13). Differential screening of a cDNA library prepared from RNA of squamous-differentiated cells resulted in the isolation of several cDNA clones, designated SQ10, SQ37, and C12 (14), that encode squamous cell–specific mRNAs. Other changes that accompany squamous differentiation are an increase in keratin 13 (K13) expression and a reduction in hyaluronidase synthesis (1,8).

ACTION OF RETINOIDS

Retinoids have been shown to be very important in maintaining the steady state of the normal tracheobronchial epithelium and to play a central role in determining whether cells follow a pathway of mucosecretory or squamous differentiation (Figure 2) (1,8). In vivo, vitamin A deficiency leads to hyperplasia and squamous metaplasia. Lungs of heavy smokers contain many foci of squamous metaplasia that can be reversed after higher intake of retinoids. Studies using in vitro cell-culture systems have confirmed the importance of retinoids in determining the pathway of differentiation in these epithelial cells. Tracheobronchial epithe-

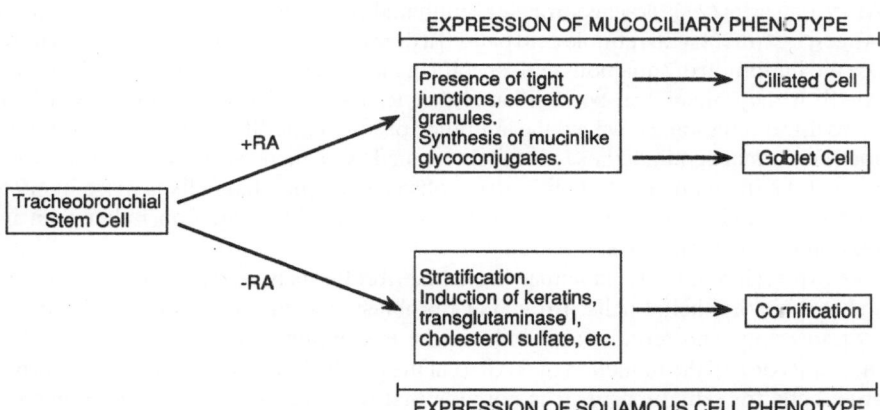

Figure 2. Central role of retinoids (RA) in the regulation of proliferation and differentiation in tracheobronchial epithelial cells. In the absence of retinoids, cells undergo squamous cell differentiation, whereas in the presence of retinoids, cells are committed to a pathway of mucociliary differentiation.

lial cells cultured in the presence of retinoids form tight junctions and secrete mucinlike glycoconjugates, whereas in the absence of retinoids, cells undergo squamous cell differentiation (15). Retinoids have been shown to inhibit the multistage process of squamous differentiation at very specific steps (8). The presence of retinoids does not prevent irreversible growth arrest when logarithmic cultures are treated with phorbol esters or interferon-γ or when cultures reach confluence. However, retinoids inhibit the induction of the squamous-differentiated phenotype as indicated by the suppression of cholesterol sulfate synthesis and by the levels of transglutaminase type I, K13, SQ10, SQ37, and C12 mRNAs (8–15).

In mammalian cells, several specific nuclear retinoic acid receptors (RARs) and cytosolic retinoic acid–binding proteins (CRABPs) have been identified (16). The RAR family consists of three different genes, designated RAR-α, RAR-β, and RAR-γ, that have a molecular weight of approximately 50,000 and are localized almost solely in the nucleus. The RARs belong to the family of steroid and thyroid hormone receptors (17). Like other members of this family, RARs contain a DNA- and ligand-binding domain (C- and E-region, respectively) and a hinge domain (D-region) that connects the DNA- and ligand-binding domains. These three domains are highly conserved among the RAR receptors. The amino-terminal (A-region) and the carboxy-terminal (F-region) domains are not very conserved among the RAR receptors. Via alternative splicing, each of the RAR genes can give rise to several transcripts that differ in their A-regions (18). It has been proposed that the A-region may be important in determining the specificity of the interaction of the RARs with other nuclear proteins thereby involved in the specificity of the transcriptional regulation by retinoic acid.

Retinoids have been shown to be able to induce, as well as inhibit, gene expression. These effects on gene expression may occur through different mechanisms. One type of regulation may occur via the classic mechanism of steroid hormone action by which transcriptional activation of certain genes appears to be mediated by specific ligand response elements (16,17). In the case of retinoic acid action, it has been suggested that binding of retinoic acid to RARs in the nucleus induces an interaction of the RAR-retinoic acid complex with specific retinoic acid response elements (RAREs) in the promoter region of responsive genes, thereby influencing their rate of transcription. Recently, one such RARE was identified in the promoter region of the RAR-β gene (19). This RARE is composed of a direct repeat of the sequence GTTCAC separated by five nucleotides. Recent evidence suggests that the binding of a RAR to a RARE may involve the formation of complexes of a RAR with other transcriptional factors (20).

To determine the mechanism of action of retinoids in tracheobronchial epithelial cells, we began to examine the expression of RARs in normal human and rabbit tracheobronchial epithelial cells. These cells express two RAR-α transcripts, 2.6 and 3.5 kb in size, and one 3.1-kb RAR-γ transcript (21). Tracheobronchial epithelial cells contained very low levels of RAR-β; however, treatment with retinoic acid caused a dramatic increase in the expression of RAR-β. Since the inhibition of squamous cell–specific genes appears to coincide with the induction of RAR-β, it may, therefore, be concluded that RAR-β is involved in the suppression of squamous differentiation. However, the inhibition of squamous differentiation by retinoic acid in human epidermal keratinocytes is not accompanied by an increase in RAR-β. Therefore, we believe that the induction of RAR-β in tracheobronchial epithelial cells is more likely to be involved in the induction of normal mucosecretory cell differentiation rather than in the suppression of squamous differentiation.

The expression of RARs in human bronchial fibroblasts is very similar to that in human tracheobronchial epithelial cells. Bronchial fibroblasts contain predominantly RAR-α and RAR-γ transcripts, and retinoic acid induces the expression of RAR-β in these cells. The presence of RAR and the induction of RAR-β in these cells indicate that bronchial fibroblasts are target cells for retinoic acid. It is possible that some of the effects of retinoids on the tracheobronchial epithelium are mediated indirectly through an action of retinoids on the bronchial fibroblasts.

Given the central role that retinoids play in controlling hyperplasia in the tracheobronchial epithelium, retinoids may be relevant to neoplasia in two major ways. First, the ability of retinoids to reverse certain hyperplastic lesions in the airways suggests that these agents may be useful in chemoprevention. Second, changes in the signal transduction pathway of retinoid action may result in aberrant control of cell growth and differentiation and contribute to the neoplastic nature of affected cells.

REFERENCES

1. Jetten AM. Growth and differentiation factors in the tracheobronchial epithelium. Am J Physiol, in press.
2. Stiles AD, D'Ercole AJ. The insulin-like growth factors and the lung. Am J Respir Cell Mol Biol 3:93–100, 1990.
3. Jetten AM, Vollberg TM, Nervi C, George MD. Positive and negative regulation of proliferation and differentiation in tracheobronchial epithelial cells. Am Rev Respir Dis 142:S36–S39, 1990.
4. Stahlman MT, Gray ME, Chytil F, Sundell H. The effect of retinol on fetal lamb tracheal epithelium with and without epidermal growth factor: A model for the effect of retinol on the healing lung of human premature infants. Lab Invest 59:25–35, 1988.
5. Finch PW, Rubin JS, Miki T, Ron D, Aaronson SA. Human KGF is FGF-related with properties of a paracrine effector of epithelial cell growth. Science 245:752–755, 1989.
6. Damstrup L, Rorth M, Skovgaard-Poulsen H. Growth factors and growth factor receptors in human malignancies, with special reference to human lung cancer: A review. Lung Cancer 5:49–68, 1989.
7. Viallet J, Minna JD. Dominant oncogenes and tumor suppressor genes in the pathogenesis of lung cancer. Am J Respir Cell Mol Biol 2:225–232, 1990.
8. Jetten AM. Multi-step process of squamous differentiation of tracheobronchial epithelial cells in vitro: Analogy with epidermal differentiation. Environ Health Perspect 80:149–160, 1989.
9. Jetten AM, Shirley JE. Characterization of transglutaminase activity in rabbit tracheal epithelial cells: Regulation by retinoids. J Biol Chem 261:15097–15101, 1986.
10. Jetten AM, George MD, Pettit GR, Rearick JI. Effects of bryostatins and retinoic acid on phorbol ester- and diacylglycerol-induced squamous differentiation in human tracheobronchial epithelial cells. Cancer Res 49:3990–3995, 1989.
11. Rearick JI, Hesterberg TW, Jetten AM. Human bronchial epithelial cells synthesize cholesterol sulfate during squamous differentiation in vitro. J Cell Physiol 133:573–578, 1987.
12. Rearick JI, Albro PW, Jetten AM. Cholesterol sulfotransferase activity is induced upon squamous differentiation of RTE cells in vitro. J Biol Chem 262:13069–13074, 1987.
13. Floyd EE, Jetten AM. Regulation of type I (epidermal) transglutaminase mRNA levels during squamous differentiation: Downregulation by retinoids. Mol Cell Biol 9:4846–4851, 1989.
14. Smits HL, Floyd EE, Jetten AM. Molecular cloning of gene sequences regulated during squamous differentiation of tracheal epithelial cells and controlled by retinoic acid. Mol Cell Biol 7:4017–4023, 1987.
15. Rearick JI, Deas MA, Jetten AM. Synthesis of mucous glycoproteins by rabbit tracheal cells in vitro. Biochem J 242:19–25, 1987.
16. Jetten AM. Regulation of gene expression by retinoic acid: Embryonal carcinoma cell differentiation. In Fisher PB (ed): Mechanisms of Differentiation, Vol. I. Boca Raton: CRC Press, 1990, pp. 49–74.
17. Evans RM. The steroid and thyroid hormone receptor superfamily. Science 240:889–895, 1988.
18. Kastner P, Krust A, Mendelsohn C, Garnier JM, Zelent A, Leroy P, Staub A, Chambon P. Murine isoforms of the retinoic acid receptor γ with specific patterns of expression. Proc Natl Acad Sci USA 87:2700–2704, 1990.
19. de The H, del Mar Vivanco-Ruiz M, Tiollais P, Stunnenberg H, Dejean A. Identification of a retinoic acid responsive element in the retinoic acid receptor β gene. Nature 343:177–180, 1990.
20. Glass CK, Devary OV, Rosenfeld MG. Multiple cell type-specific proteins differentially regulate target sequence recognition by the α retinoic acid receptor. Cell 63:729–738, 1990.
21. Nervi C, Vollberg TM, George MD, Zelent A, Chambon P, Jetten AM. Expression of nuclear retinoic acid receptors in normal tracheobronchial epithelial cells and lung carcinoma cells. Exp Cell Res, in press.

Micronuclei as Intermediate End Points in Intervention

Miriam P. Rosin

Division of Epidemiology, Biometry & Occupational Oncology
British Columbia Cancer Agency
Vancouver, British Columbia V5Z 4E6, Canada
and
Cell Biology Laboratory
School of Kinesiology
Simon Fraser University
Burnaby, British Columbia V5A 1S6, Canada

INTRODUCTION

Nearly a decade has passed since the National Academy of Sciences Committee on Diet, Nutrition and Cancer summarized the evidence for an association between dietary intake of food containing certain vitamins, micronutrients, and other components and a decrease in the development of cancer in humans (1). These observations gave rise to a thrust in research aimed at identifying the active components in foods. It also led to the design of clinical trials to evaluate the effectiveness of particular agents in reducing cancer incidence.

The need for intermediate end points that would be helpful in the design of these long-term, large-scale intervention trials is becoming increasingly apparent. Over 500 possible chemopreventive agents have been identified (2). These compounds not only differ chemically but also appear to interrupt carcinogenesis at different stages of development via biologically diverse pathways. Mechanisms are needed whereby decisions on the choice of appropriate agents, doses, and treatment schedules for specific populations can be made.

This paper presents evidence in support of the use of the micronucleus test on epithelial cells as a tissue-specific biomarker that may be of use in the design of intervention trials. Micronucleus formation is an event biologically relevant to carcinogenesis; it is a quantitative reflection of ongoing DNA damage, more specifically of chromosomal change. Recent evidence suggests that tumor formation requires the accumulation of multiple genetic changes and that different chromosomes and chromosome regions are preferentially involved in different tumors. For example, *ras* gene mutation and allelic losses on arms 5q, 17p, and 18q have been associated with colorectal cancer (3), whereas numerical aberrations in chromosomes 1, 7, 9, 11, and 17 are associated with bladder cancer (4,5). Some chromosome changes are associated with early events, such as alteration on 1p and 3p in the development of breast cancer (6); other chromosomal abnormalities appear to be associated with either progression of the disease or poor prognosis, such as alterations in 8q, 11p, 11q, 13q, and 17q in breast cancers (6) and allelic loss of chromosome 17p in bladder cancers (7). Continuous elevation

The Biology and Prevention of Aerodigestive Tract Cancers
Edited by G.R.Newell and W.K. Hong, Plenum Press, New York, 1992

of chromosomal breakage in a tissue may be associated with an elevation in risk for cancer at that site. By blocking this activity, one or more of the required genomic changes for carcinogenesis may be prevented from occurring in a tissue.

Micronucleus Frequencies in Exfoliated Cells: Studies in High-Risk Populations

Micronuclei are formed from acentric chromosomes and chromatid fragments in proliferating cells. When a cell with such chromosomal damage divides, these fragments are excluded from the main nucleus and form membrane-bound micronuclei in the daughter cell(s). The micronuclei that are detectable in exfoliated cells seem to reflect chromatid or chromosome aberrations that occurred in the proliferating basal layer of the epithelium.

Micronucleus frequencies in exfoliated cells have been validated as tissue-specific dosimeters of carcinogen exposure in humans (8–12). This validation is based on studies of individuals belonging to population groups with life-style habits associated with an elevated risk for cancer. Initial studies included the following populations of people engaged in chewing or smoking habits associated with an increased risk for oral cancer: chewers of betel quids (composed of areca nut, betel leaves, slaked lime, and sometimes tobacco) from India, Taiwan, and the Philippines; inverted smokers from India and the Philippines; snuff dippers from Canada; users of tobacco mixed with slaked lime (Kaini tobacco) from India; users of nass (a mixture of tobacco, lime, ash, and cotton oils) from Uzbekistan in the Soviet Union; and cigarette smokers plus heavy alcohol drinkers from Canada. Micronuclei frequencies were elevated in oral mucosal cells of chewers and smokers from each of these population groups. In addition, the suspected role of carcinogen damage in elevated micronucleus frequencies is further supported by studies of carcinogen dosage and cells from specific sites. For example, betel quid chewers who restrict their chewing to one side of the mouth and thus increase the exposure show the greatest elevation of micronucleus frequencies in oral mucosal cells from this site. Nass users traditionally hold the nass under the tongue, a site that shows the greatest elevation in the frequencies of micronucleated cells.

These studies have been extended by us and by others to include additional populations who are at risk for developing cancer. Participants in these trials have included individuals with an elevated risk for developing cancer because of chronic exposure to a carcinogenic mixture or the presence of premalignant lesions, or a combination of these. Various tissues have been examined in these studies: the oral cavity (13–18), the bronchial epithelium (18,19), the esophagus (20; Zaridze DG, Stich HF, and Rosin MP, unpublished data, 1985), the cervix (12,18), and the urinary bladder (12,18,21). In each case, an elevation in micronucleus frequencies was observed in the tissue at risk for developing cancer.

Chromosomal Instability as a Result of Genetic Change (Inborn or Acquired)

The amount of genomic change in a cell is dependent not only on exposure to external carcinogenic/genotoxic agents but also on the capacity of internal protective mechanisms to prevent or repair damage to the cell's genome, or both. Our understanding of the mechanisms by which genomic stability is maintained in human cells has been largely based on studies of individuals with both inborn chromosomal instability and an elevated incidence of cancer, such as patients with Bloom syndrome, ataxia-telangiectasia, Fanconi's anemia, and xeroderma pigmentosum. These syndromes, however, are rare.

It is possible that "normal" individuals belonging to the general population could acquire genomic instability in individual cells of a tissue by mutation in genetic loci responsible for the maintenance of genomic integrity. Such mutation could result from exposure to a carcinogenic agent or, alternatively, from spontaneous processes (endogenous sources of DNA damage). An elevation in genetic instability in a premalignant cell(s) would lead to an accelerated process of genetic change in a tissue, thereby increasing the probability of the cell's accumulating the multiple changes required for tumorigenesis. In support of this hypothesis are reports of an elevation in chromosomal change associated with dysplasias and carcinomas. Added support is seen in the chromosomal instability long associated with clonal expansion and neoplastic evolution.

Several of our recent studies have focused on determining whether the micronucleus test on exfoliated cells could be used to identify inborn or acquired genetic changes that result in elevated chromosomal instability. Our initial studies involving patients with Bloom syndrome, ataxia-telangiectasia, or xeroderma pigmentosum support the use of this test for such a purpose. These studies showed that micronuclei frequencies were significantly elevated above control levels in oral mucosal and urothelial cells of patients with Bloom syndrome and ataxia-telangiectasia. This elevation occurred in the absence of any known carcinogen exposure (22,23). In addition, 16 out of 26 of the examined parents of ataxia-telangiectasia patients (obligate heterozygotes) also displayed elevated micronucleus frequencies. This fact is significant since ataxia-telangiectasia heterozygotes represent up to 2.8% of the general population and have a reported elevation in cancer at a variety of epithelial sites (24,25).

In patients with xeroderma pigmentosum, the elevation in micronucleus frequencies was associated with sunlight exposure occurring primarily in cells on the dorsal tip of the tongue (8,26). These latter data are the first evidence for the interaction of genetic and environmental factors in determining micronucleus frequencies in specific tissue sites. Of interest also is the observation that among xeroderma pigmentosum patients, compared with a white (Caucasian) control population, a 20,000-fold elevation occurred in the frequency of squamous cell carcinoma on the tip of the tongue (27).

We have extended our studies on the ataxia-telangiectasia syndrome by focusing on the hypothesis that the etiology of the spontaneous chromosomal instability in these patients comes from a defect in the protection of ataxia-telangiectasia cells from reactive oxygen species (28). Table 1 presents results that support this hypothesis. Ataxia-telangiectasia cultures that are exposed to hydrogen peroxide or to a mixture of xanthine and xanthine oxidase show an elevation in micronucleus frequencies that is significantly greater than that observed in normal cultures.

Reactive oxygen species, which are generated by normal cellular respiration or during metabolism of a wide range of xenobiotics, are ubiquitous in a cell. The extent to which such species could play a role in chromosomal instability in Ataxia-telangiectasia patients or in premalignant lesions of "normal" individuals is unknown. Cells have a variety of defense mechanisms to protect them from DNA damage. These protection mechanisms include the activities of enzymes such as catalase, superoxide dismutase, and glutathione peroxidase, and the presence of cellular antioxidants, as well as the action of repair mechanisms on DNA damage to prevent it from becoming a permanent lesion. Recent reports suggest that these avenues of defense may be compromised in ataxia-telangiectasia cells. A reduction in catalase levels (30) and a defect in glutathione metabolism (31) have both been reported in ataxia-

Table 1. Sensitivity of Ataxia-Telangiectasia Cultures to Oxidative Stress

Culture	Cytokinesis-blocked Cells with Micronuclei (%)[a]		
	None	H_2O_2[b]	X/XO[b]
Ataxia-telangiectasia cultures (n = 4)	11.4	30.5	38.2
Normal cultures (n = 4)	1.2	4.7	5.3

[a]The cytokinesis-block assay of Fenech and Morley (29) was used to control for variations among cultures in toxicity and growth inhibition.
[b]H_2O_2 treatment (1 hr at 1.2 µg/ml); X/XO treatment (1 hr with 174 µg/ml xanthine and 0.05 µg/ml xanthine oxidase). $P < 0.01$ for comparison between ataxia-telangiectasia and normal cultures for spontaneous frequency, and frequencies induced by H_2O_2 and X/XO.

telangiectasia cells. Sanford and co-workers have shown that a significant elevation in chromosomal breakage occurs in ataxia-telangiectasia cells compared with normal cells after exposure to X rays during the G_2 phase (32). This response has been attributed to a defect in the capability of ataxia-telangiectasia cells to monitor and repair DNA damage in this stage of the cell cycle. It is possible that the repair of damage owing to reactive oxygen species may also be defective. Of interest are the increasing number of reports of possible defects in protection against oxidant stress in premalignant lesions such as cervical intraepithelial neoplasia and in cells from individuals from cancer-prone families (32–35). Whether these observations point to the acquisition of mutations in some premalignant lesions that make them genetically labile is yet to be determined. Also unanswered is whether chemopreventive agents could be used to suppress chromosomal instability in individuals with inborn or acquired genetic instability.

New Studies on the Role of Infections, Tissue Trauma, and Inflammatory Reactions in Chromosomal Instability and Cancer

Tissue trauma, chronic infections, and the ensuing inflammatory reactions have been associated with cancers at a variety of sites and in many populations (36–38). However, the significance of this relationship is yet to be resolved.

We have recently embarked on an international research collaboration with Dr. W. Anwar (Department of Community, Environment and Occupational Medicine, Ain Shams University, Cairo, Egypt) to study the role of inflammatory reactions in chromosomal instability and tumor promotion. The research is focused on a widespread health problem in Egypt, infection with the parasite *Schistosoma*. Worldwide, an estimated 200 million people are infected with *Schistosoma*, of which 16 species are known to infect humans or animals. Infection with two of these species (*haematobium* and *japonicum*) has been associated with an elevation in cancer in humans (39–41). The association between infection with *S. haematobium* and primary malignant disease of the urinary bladder is well documented. In areas with a high rate of infection by this species, such as Egypt, 11–44% of cancer cases are in the urinary bladder (41).

Initial studies aimed at identifying a mechanism whereby infection with *S. haematobium* could either directly or indirectly cause bladder cancer have focused on the chronic irritation and inflammation produced by the parasite eggs when they are shed into the venules of the mucosa of the bladder. These eggs either penetrate the mucosa and are released into the urine or become trapped in the tissue. A chronic inflammatory reaction is initiated with associated pathology (granuloma formation and fibrosis). In addition, ulceration and tissue damage are extensive and lead to a proliferative response and to metaplastic and dysplastic conditions.

Our first study was initiated in Fayoum Governorate in the village of Shakshouk, where the incidence of infection is approximately 40%. Urine samples were obtained from infected males 8–40 years old and from age-matched controls. Urothelial cells were collected from the urine by centrifugation. Figure 1 shows a histogram presentation of micronucleus frequencies

Figure 1. Histogram showing the distribution frequency of micronucleated cells in exfoliated urothelial cells isolated from the urine of individuals with schistosomiasis (n = 37) and age-matched controls. Means of the two populations are significantly different ($P < 0.01$) (Rosin and Anwar, unpublished data).

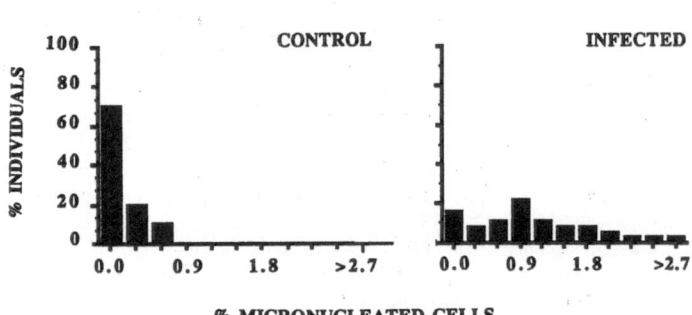

in urothelial cells from infected patients and controls. Micronucleus frequencies were significantly elevated in urothelial cells from individuals with infection ($P < 0.01$).

Support for the involvement of the schistosomal infection in this elevated chromosomal breakage comes from a recently completed pilot study in which nine infected people were treated with a single dose of the antischistosomal agent praziquantel and re-tested 6 weeks later. As shown in Figure 2, a decrease in the frequency of micronucleated cells occurred in each of these individuals, with seven patients displaying frequencies within the limits of those observed for noninfected controls. Concurrent with the reduction in micronucleus frequencies was a marked decrease in the number of inflammatory cells and the absence of eggs in urothelial sediments.

We are currently extending these studies to better define the mechanism by which infection and inflammation cause an elevation in chromosomal breakage. Recent in vitro studies suggest that the polymorphonuclear leukocytes and macrophages that infiltrate tissues during inflammation may directly damage tissue DNA through the production of reactive oxygen species. These oxygen species induce DNA strand breakage, chromosomal changes, and malignant transformation in mammalian cells cocultured with activated leukocytes (37–43). The extent to which these activities occur in vivo in humans and whether they directly contribute to an increased cancer risk are yet to be demonstrated. Other possible mechanisms whereby chromosomal breakage could be induced in patients with schistosomiasis are elevated cellular proliferation in the infected bladder, which increases DNA damage in the urothelium by reducing the time for DNA repair and leads to fixation of DNA lesions (36,44); an alteration in the activation/detoxification of carcinogenic/genotoxic agents in inflamed tissue (45); and production of nitrosamines by bacterial superinfections in the bladders of individuals with chronic schistosomiasis (41). Future studies will make use of a battery of biomarkers (micronuclei, proliferation, and metabolism markers) to explore these hypotheses. In addition, small pilot studies will be conducted with several chemopreventive regimens in an effort to suppress the chromosomal breakage in infected individuals. Treatment with antischistosomal agents has had limited success in controlling this disease in Egypt because the rate of reinfection with the parasite is very high. Alternate methods of protection, such as chemoprevention, would be greatly beneficial. Possible chemopreventive agents include antiproliferative agents (e.g., retinoids), prostaglandin synthesis inhibitors (e.g., piroxicam and aspirin), and free-radical scavengers (e.g., β-carotene and α-tocopherol).

Micronuclei as Tools for Intervention

In 1982, we proposed the possible use of micronuclei formation in exfoliated human cells as a method of estimating the efficiency of chemoprevention programs. This proposal was

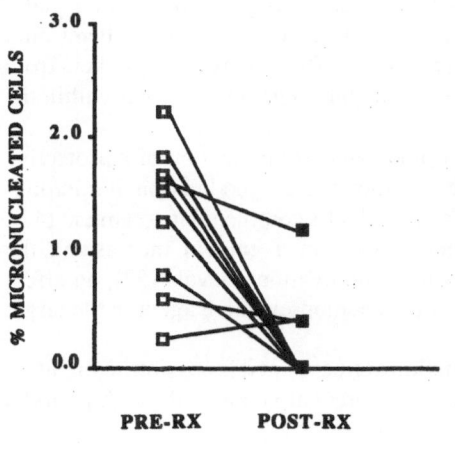

Figure 2. Changes in the frequencies of micronucleated urothelial cells in nine male patients with schistosomiasis who were treated with praziquantel (Rosin and Anwar, unpublished data).

based on two observations (46). First, we had been studying the temporal pattern of micronucleus production in cancer patients receiving radiotherapy to the head and neck region. An increase in micronucleated mucosal cells from the irradiated area occurred within 1 week of the patient's commencing treatment. The micronucleus frequency increased throughout treatment and then, within 1 month of cessation of treatment, rapidly declined to values observed in untreated tissues. This response was thought to reflect the time for cells in the basal cell layer to divide one to two times, followed by the migration of these basal cells to the surface. The second set of observations was based on the increase in micronucleated cells observed in exfoliated cell samples from the oral mucosa of betel quid chewers, snuff dippers, and users of various tobacco-containing mixtures. It was reasoned that if a chemopreventive agent was to be effective in protecting cells from genotoxic damage, the response should be quickly apparent as a reduction in micronucleus frequencies in the carcinogen-exposed tissue of such individuals.

Our first intervention trial involved a group of betel quid (areca nut, betel leaf, tobacco, and lime) chewers from northern Luzon, an island in the Philippines (47). Vitamin A (50,000 U retinyl palmitate) and β-carotene (90 mg) were administered twice weekly for 3 months. Although the participants continued chewing, a decrease in the micronucleus frequencies in the mucosal cells of the chewers became apparent within 4 weeks of treatment. After 3 months, the average frequency of micronucleated cells had fallen from 4.62% to 0.96%. Values observed in individuals receiving a placebo treatment remained unchanged.

As of this writing, several other intervention trials have been completed or initiated, their aim being to assess the response of micronucleus frequencies to various intervention regimens. These trials, which encompass studies on the oral cavity, esophagus, urinary bladder, and bronchial epithelium, involve populations from several regions of the world, including North America. Participants include people who have an elevated risk for cancer resulting from chronic exposure to a carcinogenic mixture (48–51), those who exhibit premalignant lesions (15,19,50–52), or those who belong to populations with an elevated frequency of such lesions and increased cancer incidence (13), or any combination of these.

The following observations can be drawn from these studies:

(a) The micronucleus test can be used to assess the relative efficacy of different chemopreventive regimens in providing protection against chromosomal breakage. For example, micronucleus frequencies in oral mucosal cells of betel quid chewers in the Philippines are reduced by oral supplementation with β-carotene, retinyl palmitate, or both; however, canthaxanthin supplementation is noneffective (47,48). Similarly, supplementation with folic acid (10 mg daily) does not reduce micronucleus frequencies in betel quid chewers in India, although both β-carotene and retinyl palmitate do (Stich HF and Rosin MP, unpublished data, 1985).

(b) Responses of micronucleus frequencies to a given chemopreventive regimen are population specific. For instance, β-carotene or β-carotene plus retinyl palmitate are equally effective in reducing the frequency of micronuclei in oral mucosal cells from betel quid chewers, but this treatment does not exert a chemopreventive effect in inverted smokers from Mindoro, a central island of the Philippines, who keep the burning end of a cigar within the mouth (50).

(c) Alterations in micronucleus frequencies provide an early indication of a protective effect of a chemopreventive agent in a target tissue. The quantifiable modulation of micronuclei frequencies is apparent within 1–3 months of an individual's commencing treatment (47).

(d) Cessation of a chemopreventive treatment results in a gradual increase in the frequency of micronucleated cells in the target tissue to pretreatment levels (53), an effect possibly caused by a gradual decrease in the level of the chemopreventive agent in the target tissue.

(e) Recent studies have shown that after termination of treatment it is possible to maintain a protective effect with a relatively high dose of a chemopreventive agent through periodic supplementation with lower maintenance doses (53). Giving betel quid chewers 50,000 units of retinyl palmitate per week kept micronucleus frequencies at low levels for 12 months following termination of a chemopreventive study using β-carotene (180 mg/week) and retinyl palmitate (100,000 U/week). The recurrence of elevated micronucleus frequencies and of other intermediate end points, such as leukoplakia (53), after cessation of treatment with chemopreventive agents suggests that successful chemoprevention of cancer may require continuous intake of chemopreventive agents by an individual. The possibility of giving periodic booster shots of an agent or low-dose maintenance shots thus becomes a critical issue.

Several recent chemoprevention trials have concurrently monitored the response of micronucleus frequencies and premalignant lesions (leukoplakia, dysplasia, hyperplasia) in individuals supplemented with chemopreventive agents (Table 2). Our experience is based on the responses of these two end points in chewers of tobacco-containing betel quid who are supplemented with β-carotene (180 mg/week), retinyl palmitate (100,000 U/week or 200,000 U/week), or β-carotene (180 mg/week) plus retinyl palmitate (100,000 U/week) (51–53). A reduced frequency of micronucleated mucosal cells and the remission of leukoplakias occurred with each regimen following a 3- to 6-month treatment. An inhibition in the development of new leukoplakias was also observed. However, the two end points differed in degree and in the response time required after administration of the β-carotene and retinol palmitate.

Table 2. Use of Micronucleus Test in Intervention Trials

Population	Agent	Site(s)	Micronucleus[a]	Lesion[b]	Ref. No.
Betel quid chewers	β-carotene	Oral	Decr	—	48
(India, the Philippines)	Retinyl palmitate	Oral	Decr	—	48
	β-carotene and retinyl palmitate	Oral	Decr	—	47
	Canthaxanthin	Oral	NE	—	48
Snuff users (Canada)	β-Carotene	Oral	Decr	—	49
Inverted smokers (India, the Philippines)	β-Carotene and retinyl palmitate	Oral	NE	NE	50
Betel quid chewers	β-Carotene	Oral	Decr	REM	51
(India)	β-Carotene and retinol palmitate	Oral	Decr	REM	51
	Retinyl palmitate	Oral		REM	52
	Folic acid	Oral	NE	—	c
China study[d]	Riboflavin, retinol, and zinc	Oral	NE	NE	13
		Esophagus	Decr	NE	13
S. haematobium infection (Egypt)	Praziquantel	Bladder	Decr	—	e
Oral leukoplakia (Texas)	13-cis–Retinoic acid	Oral	Decr	REM	15
Premalignant bronchial lesions (Texas)	13-cis–Retinoic acid	Bronchi	IP[d]	IP	19

Abbreviations: Decr, decrease (significant) in values; NE, no effect; IP, in progress; REM, remission of lesion
[a]Effect of treatment on micronucleus frequencies: MN, micronucleus; significant decrease in values; NE, no effect
[b]Studies in which the effect of treatment on premalignant lesions (leukoplakia, dysplasia, hyperplasia) was monitored concurrently with micronucleus frequencies.
[c]MP Rosin and HF Stich, unpublished data.
[d]Individuals randomly chosen from population in Huixian, People's Republic of China, a region with elevated incidence of esophageal cancer.
[e]MP Rosin and W Anwar, unpublished data.

All treatments were equally effective in decreasing the frequency of micronucleated cells in the oral cavities of chewers. However, treatments including retinyl palmitate were more effective in causing a reduction in leukoplakia or an inhibition of the development of new lesions. In addition, a longer supplementation time was required for changes to occur in leukoplakias (3–6 months) than the time needed for a decrease in micronucleus frequencies.

These data point to the necessity of employing a battery of end points in chemopreventive trials. Numerous changes occur in tissues during carcinogenesis. Chemoprevention agents will demonstrate specificity with respect to the particular biologic events they modulate as well as to the dose and the time required for such modulation to occur. The micronucleus test appears to be an appropriate test to include in such a battery of end points because it represents a biologically relevant end point, elevated in tissues of individuals at increased risk for cancer, and capable of being modulated by chemopreventive regimens.

ACKNOWLEDGMENTS

These studies were supported by the Natural Science and Engineering Research Council of Canada and the National Cancer Institute of Canada.

The author would like to acknowledge the technical assistance of Ms. T. MacDonald and the involvement of Ms. A.-M. Gilbert in preparation of the illustrations.

REFERENCES

1. U.S. National Research Council. Committee on Diet, Nutrition and Cancer. Diet, Nutrition and Cancer. Washington, D.C., 1982.
2. Malone WF, Kelloff GJ, Pierson H, Greenwald P. Chemoprevention of bladder cancer. Cancer 60:650–657, 1987.
3. Vogelstein B, Kern SE, Hamilton SR. Clinical implications of colorectal tumor mutations (abstract). Proceedings of the American Association for Cancer Research 31:455, 1990.
4. Hopman AHN, Moesker O, Wim A, Smeets GB, Pauwels RPE, Vooijs GP, Ramaekers FCS. Numerical chromosome 1,7,9, and 11 aberrations in bladder cancer detected by in situ hybridization. Cancer Res 51:644–651, 1991.
5. Tsai YC, Nichols PW, Hiti AL, Williams Z, Skinner DG, Jones PA. Allelic losses of chromosomes 9, 11, and 17 in human bladder cancer. Cancer Res 50:44–47, 1990.
6. Mars WM, Saunders GF. Chromosomal abnormalities in human breast cancer. Cancer and Metastasis Rev 9:35–43, 1990.
7. Olumi AF, Tsai YC, Nichols PW, Skinner DG, Cain DR, Bender LI, Jones PA. Allelic loss of chromosome 17p distinguishes high grade from low grade transitional cell carcinomas of the bladder. Cancer Res 50:7081–7083, 1990.
8. Rosin MP. Antigenotoxic action of carotenoids in carcinogen-exposed populations. Basic Life Sciences 52:45–59, 1990.
9. Rosin MP, Dunn BP, Stich HF. Use of intermediate end points in quantitating the response of precancerous lesions to chemopreventive agents. Can J Physiol Pharmacol 65:483–487, 1987.
10. Stich HF, Rosin MP. Micronuclei in exfoliated human cells as a tool for studies in cancer risk and cancer intervention. Cancer Lett 22:241–253, 1984.
11. Stich HF, Rosin MP. Quantitating the synergistic effect of smoking and alcohol consumption with the micronucleus test on human buccal mucosa cells. Int J Cancer 31:305–308, 1983.
12. Stich HF. Micronucleated cells as indicators for genotoxic damage and as markers in chemoprevention trials. Journal of Nutrition, Growth and Cancer 4:9–18, 1987.
13. Munoz N, Hayashi M, Lu JB, Wahrendorf J, Crespi M, Bosch FX. Effect of riboflavin, retinol, and zinc on micronuclei of buccal mucosa and of esophagus: A randomized double-blind intervention study in China. J Natl Cancer Inst 79:687–691, 1987.
14. Lippman SM, Lee JS, Lotan R, Hittelman W, Wargovich MJ, Hong WK. Biomarkers as intermediate end points in chemoprevention trials. J Natl Cancer Inst 82:555–560, 1990.
15. Lippman SM, Toth BB, Batsakis JG, Weber RS, McCarthy KS, Hays GL, Wargovich MJ, Lee JS, Thacher S, Lotan R. Modulation by 13-*cis* retinoic acid of biologic markers as indicators of intermediate end points in human

oral carcinogenesis. Prog Clin Biol Res 339:179–191, 1990.

16. Picker JD, Fox DP. Do curried foods produce micronuclei in buccal epithelial cells? Mutat Res 171:185–188, 1986.

17. Livingston GK, Reed RN, Olson BL, Lockey JE. Induction of nuclear aberrations by smokeless tobacco in epithelial cells of human oral mucosa. Environ Mol Mutagen 15:136–144, 1990.

18. Fontham E, Correa P, Rodriguez E, Lin Y. Validation of smoking history with the micronuclei test. In Hoffmann D, Harris CC (eds): Mechanisms in Tobacco Carcinogenesis. Cold Spring Harbor, NY: Cold Spring Harbor Laboratory, 1986, pp. 113–119.

19. Lippman SM, Peters EJ, Wargovich MJ, Stadnyk AN, Dixon DO, Dekmezian RH, Loewy JW, Morice RC, Cunningham JE, Hong WK. Bronchial micronuclei as a marker of an early stage of carcinogenesis in the human tracheobronchial epithelium. Int J Cancer 45:811–815, 1990.

20. Mandard AM, Duigou F, Marnay J, Masson P, Qiu SL, Yi JS, Barrellier P, Lebigot G. Analysis of the results of the micronucleus test in patients presenting upper digestive tract cancers and in non-cancerous subjects. Int J Cancer 39:442–444, 1987.

21. Reali D, DiMarino F, Bahramandpour S, Carducci A, Barale R, Loprieno N. Micronuclei in exfoliated urothelial cells and urine mutagenicity in smokers. Mutat Res 192:145–149, 1987.

22. Rosin MP, German J. Evidence for chromosomal instability in vivo in Bloom syndrome: Increased number of micronuclei in exfoliated cells. Hum Genet 71:187–191, 1985.

23. Rosin MP, Ochs HD, Gatti RA, Boder E. Heterogeneity of chromosomal breakage levels in epithelial tissue of ataxia-telangiectasia homozygotes and heterozygotes. Hum Genet 83:133–138, 1989.

24. Swift M, Morrell D, Cromartie E, Chamberlin AR, Skolnick MH, Bishop DT. The incidence and gene frequency of ataxia-telangiectasia in the United States. Am J Hum Genet 39:573–583, 1986.

25. Swift M, Chase CL, Morrell D. Cancer predisposition of ataxia-telangiectasia heterozygotes. Cancer Genetics and Cytogenetics 46:21–27, 1990.

26. Rosin MP, Gilbert A-M. Modulation of genotoxic effects in humans. In Mendelsohn ML, Albertini RJ (eds): Mutation and the Environment, Part E: Environmental Genotoxicity, Risk, and Modulation. New York: Wiley-Liss, 1990, pp. 351–360.

27. Keukens F, Van Voorst Vader PC, Panders AK, Vinks S, Oosterhuis JW, Kleijer WJ. Xeroderma pigmentosum: Squamous cell carcinoma of the tongue. Acta Derm Venereol (Stockh) 69:530–531, 1989.

28. Yi M, Rosin MP, Anderson CK. Response of fibroblast cultures from ataxia-telangiectasia patients to oxidative stress. Cancer Lett 54:43–50, 1990.

29. Fenech M, Morley AA. Measurement of micronuclei in lymphocytes. Mutat Res 147:29–36, 1985.

30. Vuillaume M. Reduced oxygen species, mutation, induction and cancer initiation. Mutat Res 186:43–72, 1987.

31. Meredith MM, Dodson M. Impaired glutathione biosynthesis in cultured human ataxia-telangiectasia cells. Cancer Res 47:4576–4581, 1987.

32. Sanford KK, Parshad R, Gantt R, Tarone RE, Jones GM, Price FM. Factors affecting and significance of G_2 chromatin radiosensitivity in predisposition to cancer. Int J Radiat Biol 55:963–981, 1989.

33. Benedetto C, Bajardi F, Ghiringhello B, Marozio L, Nohammer G, Phitakpraiwan P, Rojanapo W, Schauenstein E, Slater TF. Quantitative measurements of the changes in protein thiols in cervical intraepithelial neoplasia and in carcinoma of the human uterine cervix provide evidence for the existence of a biochemical field effect. Cancer Res 50:6663–6667, 1990.

34. Rabilloud T, Asselineau D, Miquel C, Calvayrac R, Darmon M, Vuillaume M. Deficiency in catalase activity correlates with the appearance of tumor phenotype in human keratinocytes. Int J Cancer 45:952–956, 1990.

35. Vuillaume M, Decroix Y, Truc JB, Paniel BJ, Calvayrac R, Hubert M, Poitout P. Deficiency in the catalase activity of human cervical intraepithelial neoplasia, immediately adjacent tissues and early invasive neoplasia. Cancer (in press).

36. Preston-Martin S, Pike MC, Ross RK, Jones PA, Henderson BE. Increased cell division as a cause of human cancer. Cancer Res 50:7415–7421, 1990.

37. Gordon LI, Weitzman SA. The respiratory burst and carcinogenesis. In Sbarra AJ, Strauss RR (eds): The Respiratory Burst and Its Physiological Significance. New York: Plenum Publishing, 1988, pp. 277–298.

38. Kaplan RP. Cancer complicating chronic ulcerative and scarifying mucocutaneous disorders. Adv Dermatol 2:19–46, 1987.

39. Chen M, Mott K. Progress in assessment of morbidity due to *Schistosoma haematobium* infection. Tropical Diseases Bulletin 86:2–36, 1989.

40. Chen M, Mott K. Progress in assessment of morbidity due to *Schistosoma japonicum* infection. Tropical Diseases Bulletin 85:2–56, 1988.

41. Tawfik HN. Carcinoma of the urinary bladder associated with schistosomiasis in Egypt: The possible causal relationship. In Miller RW (ed): Unusual Occurrences As Clues to Cancer Etiology. Tokyo Japan Scientific Societies Press, 1988, pp. 197–209.

42. Cerutti P. Prooxidant states and tumor promotion. Science 227:375–381, 1985.

43. Kensler TW, Egner PA, Taffe BG, Trush MA. Role of free radicals in tumor promotion and progression. In Slaga TJ, Klein-Szanto AJP, Boutwell RK, Stevenson DE, Spitzer HL, D'Motto B (eds): Skin Carcinogenesis: Mechanisms and Human Relevance. New York: Alan R. Liss, 1989, pp. 233–248.

44. Ames BN, Gold LS. Too many rodent carcinogens: Mitogenesis increases mutagenesis. Science 249:970–971, 1990.

45. Eling TE, Thompson DC, Foureman GL, Curtis JF, Hughes MF. Prostaglandin H synthase and xenobiotic oxidation. Annual Review of Pharmacology and Toxicology 30:1–45, 1990.

46. Rosin MP, Stich HF. The identification of antigenotoxic/anticarcinogenic agents in food. In Roe DA (ed): Diet, Nutrition and Cancer: From Basic Research to Policy Implications. New York: Alan R. Liss, 1983, pp. 141–154.

47. Stich HF, Rosin MP, Vallejera MO. Reduction with vitamin A and beta-carotene administration of proportion of micronucleated buccal mucosal cells in Asian betel nut and tobacco chewers. Lancet 1:1204–1206, 1984.

48. Stich HF, Stich W, Rosin MP, Vallejera MO. Use of the micronucleus test to monitor the effect of vitamin A, beta-carotene and canthaxanthin on the buccal mucosa of betel nut/tobacco chewers. Int J Cancer 34:745–750, 1984.

49. Stich HF, Hornby AP, Dunn BP. A pilot beta-carotene intervention trial with Inuits using smokeless tobacco. Int J Cancer 36:321–327, 1985.

50. Stich HF, Rosin MP, Hornby AP, Mathew B, Sankaranarayanan R, Nair MK. Pilot intervention studies with carotenoids. In Krinsky NI, Mathews-Roth MM, Taylor RF (eds): Carotenoids: Chemistry and Biology. New York: Plenum Publishing, 1990, pp. 313–321.

51. Stich HF, Rosin MP, Hornby AP, Mathew B, Sankaranarayanan R, Nair MK. Remission of oral leukoplakias and micronuclei in tobacco/betel quid chewers treated with beta-carotene and with beta-carotene plus vitamin A. Int J Cancer 42:195–199, 1988.

52. Stich HF, Hornby AP, Mathew B, Sankaranarayanan R, Nair MK. Response of oral leukoplakias to the administration of vitamin A. Cancer Lett 40:93–101, 1988.

53. Stich HF, Mathew B, Sankaranarayanan R, Krishnan Nair M. Remission of oral precancerous lesions of tobacco/areca nut chewers following administration of beta-carotene or vitamin A, and maintenance of the protective effect. Cancer Detect Prev (in press).

Study Design for the Prevention of Aerodigestive Tract Cancers

Thomas E. Moon

Department of Family and Community Medicine
University of Arizona
Tucson, Arizona

INTRODUCTION

The randomized, double-blind clinical trial design has been regarded as the best method to evaluate a new treatment or intervention versus a control among human subjects. Such a design is not always achievable, often because of ethics. For example, in cancer etiology studies, the random allocation of an alleged carcinogen to human subjects would not be considered ethical. For this reason, use of an observational case-control or cohort study design is most commonly used in cancer epidemiology studies. In cancer therapy research, use of the randomized clinical trial design has been used for approximately 40 years. Design of aerodigestive tract cancer prevention trials, when contrasted with cancer therapy trials, requires modification of some key aspects related to methods, logistics, and cost. Many of these modifications have previously been identified by colleagues in their conduct of cardiovascular disease prevention trials (1).

SUBJECTS, NOT PATIENTS

Identification and recruitment of subjects for aerodigestive tract cancer prevention trials need to emphasize the nonclinical and free-living characteristics of study subjects. Trial designs that focus on prevention of a second aerodigestive tract cancer will commonly enroll subjects who have completed their cancer treatment and thus are undergoing only occasional clinical follow-up. Also, trials designed to prevent the initial diagnosis of cancer may enroll "high-risk" subjects. However, even high-risk subjects are uncommonly under frequent clinical follow-up before being enrolled on an aerodigestive tract cancer prevention trial. Thus, most enrolled subjects are likely to accept minimal side effects and minimal proscribed logistical conflicts in their life-style. Unacceptable side effects or life-style conflicts will lower adherence, limit subject follow-up, and reduce the number of end points as well as the statistical power of the trial.

The Biology and Prevention of Aerodigestive Tract Cancers
Edited by G.R.Newell and W.K. Hong, Plenum Press, New York, 1992

105

WHICH INTERVENTION?

Selection of the intervention should optimally be based upon a full consideration of epidemiologic and laboratory-based literature plus their conceptual interrelationship with the carcinogenesis process. Modifying the prior discussions of Byar (2) and Bertram and colleagues (3), Figure 1 shows such a conceptual interrelationship and emphasizes that cancer prevention trials may be classified in a series of five stages: Stage 1 if the intervention precedes initiation of carcinogenesis, Stage 2 or Stage 3 if the intervention impacts the promotion or progression stages of carcinogenesis, Stage 4 if the intervention impacts preneoplasia, and Stage 5 if the intervention is for treatment of neoplasia.

The selection of an intervention for a cancer prevention trial would optimally be related to environmental exposures identified by epidemiologic research, systemic or tissue-specific biochemical changes, and corresponding molecular changes. Different stages of the carcinogenic process will likely be associated with different environmental exposures, such as biochemical and molecular changes. For example, initiation of several aerodigestive tract cancers has been associated with cigarette smoking. While the factors responsible for and biomarkers of promotion and progression are not fully identified, hypotheses related to nutritional status, such as decreased carotenoids or other antioxidants, have been proposed as the exposures associated with promotion or progression. Other changes in nutritional status, such as a deficiency in cell differentiation associated with low vitamin A concentrations in tissues or increased oxidative stress, may be key exposures associated with the preneoplasia stage.

One interpretation of the conceptual framework shown in Figure 1 is that the selection of the intervention must correspond with the stage of carcinogenesis. For example, an intervention that has its maximal preventive effect only during the initiation of carcinogenesis would rarely be able to be evaluated as effective if subjects were selected exclusively from those at the preneoplasia stage. Such an intervention would act too early in the carcinogenesis process.

Use of the factorial design for simultaneously testing multiple interventions has been proposed (2). Such a design has clear sample-size advantages. Evaluating two statistically independent and biologically different interventions can be carried out with the same sample size that would be required to evaluate one intervention alone. Possibly more important is the ability of a factorial design to evaluate the biologic interrelationship between interventions. For example, the simultaneous evaluation of a retinoid and β-carotene in the prevention of aerodigestive tract cancers would provide unique information that could not be obtained by studying each agent in separate trials. Subjects assigned to receive both a retinoid and a β-carotene would provide an indication of the degree of additive or even synergistic effect of both agents combined. Although the sample size would be increased for adequate evaluation of such an interaction effect, the importance to cancer prevention research and the design of next-generation multiagent intervention trials would be substantial. The work reported by Moon

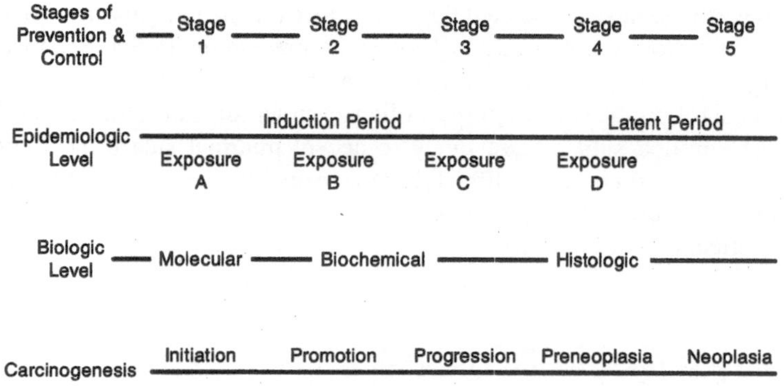

Figure 1. Relationship between stages of cancer prevention trials, epidemiology, biology, and carcinogenesis.

and colleagues (4), as part of this conference, provides an animal model that indicates a positive interaction when two agents are combined.

How Big an Effect?

Few interventions in public health have achieved a 50% or greater effect in reducing disease risk. Even a 10–20% reduction in cancer risk is meaningful for many cancers, such as colon, breast, and lung. To identify a 10–20% intervention effect, the sample size must be substantially larger than a 50% effect. A clear, yet unmet, need for conducting pilot trials before the main intervention trial is to provide an estimate of the magnitude of the intervention effect. Referred to as Phase II trials in cancer therapy, use of the diagnosis of cancer as the primary end point for current prevention trials has generally precluded use of pilot (Phase II) trials in cancer prevention. The low annual incidence of cancer and its long induction period are the primary reasons that such pilot trials have not been widely used in cancer prevention. The current unavailability of short-term, intermediate biochemical markers that can serve as a surrogate, but biologically meaningful, end point has been a major limitation in the design and conduct of cancer prevention trials. Such biomarkers would certainly facilitate both the continued integration of epidemiologic and laboratory research and the improved selection of interventions to be evaluated in a randomized cancer prevention trial.

ADHERENCE TO INTERVENTION

The safety and acceptability of an intervention to study subjects are important considerations in the design of aerodigestive tract cancer prevention trials. Decreased adherence related to intervention safety or acceptability will substantially decrease the statistical power or confidence of correctly identifying a reduction in cancer incidence among those receiving the active intervention (5). For example, a sample size of 2166 subjects, when there is 100% adherence to the protocol, may be required to evaluate a retinoid versus a placebo in the prevention of aerodigestive tract cancers. The sample size would be increased by nearly 25%, to a total of 2696 subjects, when adherence is 90%. Commonly, a 75% or lower 5-year adherence may be observed. Trials with a 75% adherence would require an increase in sample size from 2166 to a total of 4030 subjects. The efficiency and cost reduction associated with increased adherence is thus substantial.

Delayed Intervention Effect

The requisite sample size for a cancer prevention trial must be increased, to reflect a delay in the maximal intervention effect. For example, enrolled subjects who have recently been initiated by an exposure to a carcinogen may not show maximal or even any reduction in cancer risk if the intervention selected has its maximal effect during the preneoplastic stage of carcinogenesis. Using the above example, a sample size of 2166 subjects, who have immediate maximal intervention effect, has to be increased according to the proportion of the trial follow-up for which the intervention actually would be effective (5). An intervention that is effective during 90% of the study follow-up would require an approximate 25% increase in sample size, or a total of 2732 study subjects. Interventions that are maximally effective during 60% of the study follow-up only would require substantial increases in study subjects to 6530 subjects.

Who Should Be Randomized

In designing an aerodigestive tract cancer prevention trial, the question is not whether the subjects should be randomly allocated to the active versus control (placebo) intervention, but whether the randomization unit should be the individual or the community. The majority of cancer prevention trials that are currently under way have allocated individuals to the intervention. However, as cancer prevention trials progress through the phases of cancer control (6), use of communities as the unit of randomization may be the most efficient and scientifically relevant for the conduct of Phase V or demonstration trials.

Use of a run-in period to exclude those who do not adhere to individually randomized prevention trials has been generally accepted as a logistically effective and cost-effective method. The length of the run-in period has varied from 1 to as many as 6 months. Figure 2 shows the impact of a run-in period comparing 3 versus 5 months run-in for an ongoing study of retinol versus placebo in the chemoprevention of skin cancer currently under way at the University of Arizona in Tucson (T. E. Moon, 1990, written communication). After 36 months of follow-up, there are nearly identical proportions of subjects adhering to the protocol. Thus, the 5-month run-in period, which was initially chosen because of logistic considerations, was no better than a 3-month run-in period. The use of less than 3 months for a run-in period, especially a 1-month run-in, has not been fully evaluated. Based upon experience with the above-mentioned skin cancer prevention trial, a 1-month run-in period would not appear to eliminate adequately those who did not comply during the run-in.

How Many Subjects?

Cancer prevention trials generally require 10–100 times more study subjects than has been commonly included in cancer therapy trials. For example, 16,000 women have been proposed for the developing tamoxifen primary breast cancer prevention trial (Demets, 1990, written communication). A balance between the cancer risk of study subjects and the sample size is another consideration in designing a cancer prevention trial. A key question to ask is whether predominantly high-risk versus average-risk subjects should be included. Even if etiologic factors to identify high-risk subjects were fully available for aerodigestive tract cancers, the selection of the intervention would influence the risk profile of subjects and, subsequently, the number of subjects required. Interventions that are predominantly effective in the late promotional or preneoplasia stages of carcinogenesis may be evaluated in high-risk subjects using currently available epidemiologic and laboratory-identified reports of risk factors. However, a balanced view, which considers selection of an intervention and sample size, may be especially important in the evaluation of interventions that are hypothesized to

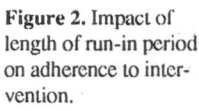

Figure 2. Impact of length of run-in period on adherence to intervention.

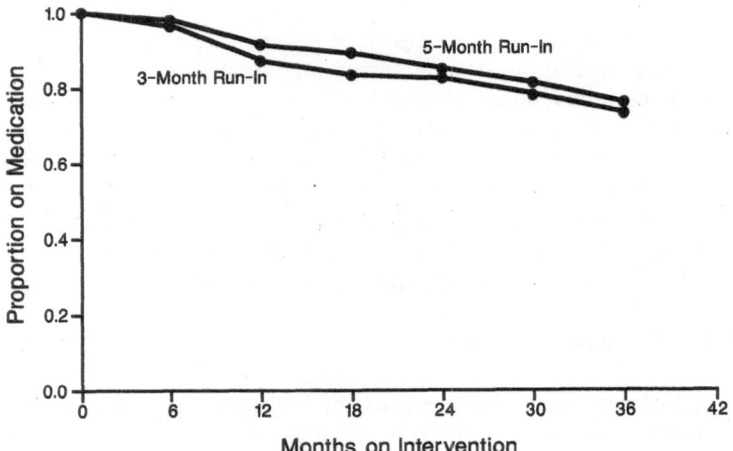

act during the promotion and progression stages of carcinogenesis. The current limitation of epidemiologic and laboratory-identified risk factors for these stages of carcinogenesis necessitate a more average-risk subject population and thus a larger sample size.

How to Monitor and Analyze the Prevention Trial

Use of a vanguard (group) has generally been successful in evaluating recruitment, safety, and process logistics for the conduct of cancer prevention trials. An unresolved question is how long one should wait before initiating the entire intervention trial to permit an adequate assessment of long-term safety and adherence before exposing large numbers of subjects to the intervention.

There are adequate statistical methods for the analysis of cancer prevention trials. The generally accepted philosophy "once randomized, always analyzed" indicates that all subjects randomized be included in the evaluation of the intervention effectiveness. A cost-effective method has been proposed by Prentice and colleagues to use a nested case-cohort methodology by which all subjects obtaining a primary end point and only a portion of other subjects will be included in the analysis of study end points and monitoring procedures (7).

CONCLUSION

There are a number of differences between prevention and treatment trials in their design, conduct, and analysis. These include the use of both epidemiologic and laboratory rationales for the trial, the number of study subjects, the selection and type of interventions, and the sample size. A substantial increase in the number of study subjects and the corresponding long duration of cancer prevention trials results in substantial cost to initiate and carry out such trials adequately. A balanced perspective of the role of cancer prevention trials would indicate that even though study duration and costs are substantial, the continued initiation of cancer prevention trials is required. The identification and validation of intermediate biochemical markers for subjects' cancer risk and intermediate end points would have substantial beneficial impact upon the cost and the number of trials that will be initiated. The use of biochemical markers would also facilitate improved cost-effective screening of potential cancer prevention agents through pilot trials.

REFERENCES

1. Halperin M, Rogot E, Gurian J, Ederer F. Sample size for medical trials with special reference to long-term therapy. Journal of Chronic Disease 21:13–24, 1968.
2. Byar DP. Some statistical considerations for design of cancer prevention trials. Prev Med 18:688–699, 1989.
3. Bertram JS, Kolonel LN, Meyskens FL. Rationale and strategies for chemoprevention of cancer in humans. Cancer Res 4:3012–3031, 1987.
4. Moon RC, Rao KVN, Detrisac CJ, Kelloff GJ. Hamster lung cancer model of carcinogenesis and chemoprevention. In Newell GR, Hong WK (eds): The Biology and Prevention of Aerodigestive Tract Cancers. New York: Plenum Publishing, 1991, pp. 55–61.
5. Moon TE. Clinical trials of cancer prevention agents: True versus observed prevention effect. Stat Med 5:435–439, 1986.
6. Greenwald P, Cullen JW. The new emphasis in cancer control. J Natl Cancer Inst 74:543–551, 1985.
7. Prentice RL. A case-cohort design for epidemiologic cohort studies and disease prevention trials. Biometrika 73:1–11, 1986.

Participant Enrollment, Participation, and Compliance in Chemoprevention Trials

Barbara K. Rimer

*Fox Chase Cancer Center
Cheltenham, Pennsylvania*

Until recently, efforts at cancer prevention were limited primarily to smoking cessation and the avoidance of occupational exposure to carcinogens. Today, these efforts have expanded to include not only dietary modification for the prevention of breast and colon cancers but also treatments with a wide array of chemopreventive agents.

Chemoprevention, defined as "the use of a pharmacologic or dietary compound to block or inhibit the development of a cancer from normal or preneoplastic tissue" (1), is linked with biology, epidemiology, and—not surprisingly—the behavioral sciences. The beliefs, knowledge, and behaviors of participants in trials involving chemoprevention and risk reduction are important considerations in planning and carrying out successful studies. In risk reduction trials, for example, potential participants must first be convinced that taking part is worth the effort. They must be motivated to adhere to the trial for a long time, perhaps indefinitely (2). Participants must also believe that the inconveniences, side effects, and costs of a study will not overshadow the benefits. If the only obvious benefit to participation is the possible avoidance of a cancer that might not develop anyway, participants may need to be shown other, more tangible benefits (3), such as weight loss through participation in a low-fat dietary trial (4). Finally, participants need to feel valued by the study team; the team's attention to building rapport and providing emotional support is especially important in long-term trials. Given the proper support by the team, people will often participate for altruistic reasons as well as for the tangible benefits they can receive (5).

Indeed, without the support of the people who have volunteered to take part, a trial is doomed before it starts. According to Levanthal et al., "The goals of participants are a source of variance that can affect recruitment, response to randomization, adherence to various components of trial protocols, and disease detection" (6). Adherence, the theme underlying all aspects of participation, is a complex dynamic phenomenon that can change over time (7) yet, as Epstein and Cluss (8) noted, is a direct influence on the effectiveness of a treatment.

*Current address: Cancer Control Research Program, Duke Comprehensive Cancer Center, Box 2949, Duke University Medical Center, Durham, NC 27710.

The Biology and Prevention of Aerodigestive Tract Cancers
Edited by G.R.Newell and W.K. Hong, Plenum Press, New York, 1992

111

RECRUITMENT

Before adherence becomes an issue, however, participants must be recruited. Because prevention trials often require large numbers of subjects for adequate statistical power, failure to recruit a large enough group can jeopardize the significance of the outcome (9–11). When a chemoprevention study requires that healthy members of the public be screened for a potentially premalignant disorder (5) or that they participate in a prolonged trial, recruitment becomes especially difficult. The ideal people to recruit for these trials, according to Stevens et al. (12), are those with the following characteristics:

- They are in good health and are able to comply physically with the demands of the trial.
- They are socially connected (i.e., they live with a spouse or family and are unlikely to leave the area).
- They are knowledgeable about the trial.
- They are motivated, at least in part, by altruism.
- They are willing to forego an intervention, if so assigned, and are willing to take a placebo.

A particular study will, to some extent, have its own participant profile. Miller et al. (13), for example, compared the characteristics of 61 participants and 28 nonparticipants in a chemoprevention trial for familial polyposis patients. Participants were younger, more recently diagnosed, more likely to be Catholic, and located farther from the trial site. They were also more likely to be happy with their marriages and to have scored at either extreme on a happiness scale used to test potential participants.

Various strategies have been used for recruitment in chemoprevention and other types of trials. Whereas several modalities have proved useful, some are more effective than others (14). Promising methods include advertising and publishing articles in the mass media, targeting specific geographic areas and worksites, using direct mail, communicating with health professional groups, soliciting through patient data bases, and identifying at-risk people through listings such as tumor registries.

ELIGIBILITY AND ENROLLMENT

Once people have been recruited to a prevention trial, the next goal is to enroll them. The study team must first assess their eligibility in relation to the goals of the trial and the treatment criteria specified in the protocol. The evidence (5) suggests that only a small proportion of those who are recruited will meet a trial's eligibility criteria. For example, in a study of the effects of tamoxifen on breast cancer risk, only 12% of the women recruited actually enrolled in the trial. Many of these were not eligible, for reasons including a wide variety of socio-demographic and health-related factors. Some did not meet the age criteria; others had health conditions that made them ineligible (15).

After eligibility is established, a large proportion of potential participants fail to enroll or participate. For example, Stevens et al. (12) estimated that only half of the respondents eligible for their skin cancer prevention and polyp trials actually enrolled. Some, for example, found the expectations for participation too great. This failure can occur for a number of reasons. Ho et al. (16) questioned people in a retirement community about participating in a study on fiber intake. Those who did not participate cited lack of interest, lack of belief in the scientific evidence, inconvenience, age, and health barriers. Sometimes enrollees have inappropriate expectations about a trial. In a study of the effects of vitamin A on lung cancer risk, for example, many of the people who initially expressed interest in participating were actually looking for a smoking cessation program (5). Others may find the activities inconvenient. In a fat-reduction trial (17), 21% of those who were enrolled dropped out after the randomization process but before intervention. When those who remained were told to keep dietary records and appointments, the participation rate further declined to 10.4%.

Occasionally, people who are excellent candidates for a study respond and enroll, only to drop out after being asked to give their informed consent. Obtaining informed consent is required by the U.S. Department of Health and Human Services for all trials funded by the government. According to the data, many of those chosen for participation in prevention trials do not give their written consent to participate. In the tamoxifen trial mentioned above, for example, although 47% of the eligible participants enrolled, 23% dropped out when asked to give their consent (15). Participants are sometimes eliminated during the run-in period required in most chemoprevention trials. For example, during the early phase of a cervical cancer chemoprevention trial, Romney et al. (18) excluded patients thought to be unreliable or potentially noncompliant. Noncompliance was also the reason physicians were dropped from the Physicians' Health Trial (19). Without effective screening to eliminate poorly motivated or ineligible participants who would drop out of a study during its later phases, a statistical bias may be established that would indicate artificially high levels of compliance and would ultimately limit the external validity of the results of a trial (5,17,18–24).

PARTICIPANT ADHERENCE

Indeed, one of the most challenging aspects of conducting prevention trials aimed at behavior change is participant adherence (often referred to in the literature as compliance). Motivating people to make long-term, sometimes lifelong, changes in habits related to diet, alcohol, or smoking requires a major commitment. Whereas the literature on participant compliance is extensive, there is still little reported experience related to chemoprevention trials (5,17,18–24).

STRATEGIES FOR IMPROVING COMPLIANCE

Before planning a chemoprevention trial, investigators should carefully examine all the elements of adherence associated with the trial. Compliance is lower, for example, when participants do not have the information or special skills needed for a study (25). It also tends to be lower with trial regimens that are longer and more complex (26,27); thus, an important concern of investigators should be the simplification of a regimen. Examiners should carefully study these requirements and other possible problems. By understanding all aspects of potential nonadherence, they can better tailor their strategies for enhancing participant cooperation. The information that follows addresses some of the strategies researchers have found that motivate trial participants and enhance a study's chance of successful completion.

Improving the Participant-Researcher Relationship

A substantial literature attests to the importance of the patient-physician relationship in facilitating adherence (28). Berenson et al. (22) highlighted the importance of trust, rapport, and integrity between the participant and study team in a fiber supplement trial for polyposis patients. Loescher et al. (29) concluded that many of their participants remained in the chemoprevention study because they liked the study team. Romney et al. (18) suggested that later recruits into their *cis*-retinol trial for the prevention of cervical cancer complied better than did earlier recruits because the former had greater rapport with their study team and "were often willing to complete their participation in spite of the difficulties and discomforts encountered." Gritz et al. (14) stressed the quality of the practitioner-client relationship as a primary ingredient in therapeutic change. They concluded that both the verbal and nonverbal communication of caring and warmth can improve rapport. Active collaboration is also facilitated when the investigators encourage and answer patient questions, when they are friendly rather than businesslike, and when they avoid medical jargon (7).

Increasing Knowledge and Skills of Participants

Understanding what to do and having the right skills to follow through are important elements of participant adherence (25). People sometimes fail to complete a trial simply because they did not understand what was expected of them (29). Helping them comprehend the regimen is an important first step. For example, one-on-one counseling by a nutritionist may be essential when asking people to make dietary changes (30). Written directions should supplement verbal discussions, and key points should be repeated. Written instructions (25,31) can have a more sustained impact on both knowledge and behavior. Attention to several communication techniques can help improve comprehension. Ley (32) has shown, for instance, that it is helpful to simplify technical information and to organize it so that the most important part is first or last.

Modifying Behaviors

Behavior modification strategies borrowed from programs ranging from weight loss to smoking cessation offer a number of practical applications for enhancing adherence. These include asking the patient to set specific goals, sign contracts, and keep records (3,14,33). Turk et al. (33) recommended contingency contracting as an especially effective means of producing initial adherence. For example, a written contract would be signed between the participant and the study team. After that, the emphasis can be shifted to more intrinsic motivations.

Enhancing Memory

Reminder and cues, such as medication timers, special calendars, and reminder letters and phone calls can help improve compliance. Evidence from various trials suggests that simplifying a regimen, such as once-a-day dosing, greatly enhances long-term compliance (34,35), as does providing devices like a calendar pack for medications.

Enhancing Problem-solving Skills

Another strategy for motivating long-term adherence is to engage participants in active problem solving to help them overcome obstacles to adherence. Asking participants to model recommended behavior is a first step. For example, a woman may decide she cannot adhere to a low-fat diet because the regimen is boring. A demonstration and sampling of appetizing, easy-to-make, low-fat foods could help reaffirm her commitment to the trial. We have used telephone counselors to make brief calls to people eligible for screening to help them identify their personal barriers and develop a plan to overcome them; after being called, 38% of the previously nonadherent women adhered to the recommended behavior (36).

Providing Tangible Support

Some people, especially poorer and older people, may fail to adhere to a regimen because they lack transportation to the trial location or money for overnight lodging or because the hours are incompatible with their schedules. Providing transportation, lodging expenses, and flexible hours may help decrease barriers to participation (37). Loescher et al. (29) asked women what changes would make it easier for them to participate in a chemoprevention trial; 27% responded "more flexible scheduling," and 8% said "provide transportation." For some populations especially, these tangible supports may be needed.

Enhancing Social Support

There is evidence that people often find it easier to change behaviors and adhere to regimens when others around them are supportive of their efforts (25,38). Acceptance of dietary change, for example, often requires family support (4). Berenson et al. (22) found better compliance for a high-fiber diet trial when a participant's breakfast was prepared by a family member. Family support, however, may not always be useful; it is probably most helpful when family members have been shown the appropriate behavior.

Improving Long-term Motivation

There is evidence that adherence deteriorates over time (5,39), so it is necessary to keep a constant vigil and plan ways to maintain the commitment of participants over time. Because prevention trials sometimes last for long periods—sometimes 5 years or more—special attention must be given to participant motivation. Positive reinforcement and feedback from the study team are essential (40). At every contact, participants should be asked how they are doing and whether they need help in overcoming any specific barriers. Occasional meetings and brief counselor contact in self-help programs (41–45) improve both adherence and outcomes. Providing toll-free telephone numbers and stamped, self-addressed cards and mailing regular reminders also aid in maintaining the cooperation required in prevention trials. Birthday and holiday cards, personalized letters, tip sheets, and newsletters (e.g., with tips on special regimens or on health care for the elderly) are useful. Small gifts, lottery prizes, and other incentives can help increase the motivation for compliance (12,41).

SUMMARY

Chemoprevention trials offer exciting opportunities for decreasing the risk for cancer. Close attention to the recruitment, enrollment, and compliance of participants will aid greatly in both the cooperation of participants and the long-term adherence that are essential for the success of these trials.

ACKNOWLEDGMENTS

This work was supported by the National Institutes of Health grant CA-34856, institutional Grants NIH CA-06927 and RR-05895 awarded to Fox Chase Cancer Center, and an appropriation from the Commonwealth of Pennsylvania.

This paper is a revised version of B. K. Rimer and P. F. Engstrom. Participation in macronutrient trials. In Micozzi M and Moon T (eds). Nutrition and Cancer Prevention: Investigating the Role of Macronutrients. New York: Marcel Dekker, in press. Copyright permission obtained from Marcel Dekker, Inc.

REFERENCES

1. Meyskens FL Jr. The place of chemoprevention studies in cancer prevention planning. In Mettlin CJ, Aoki K (eds): Recent Progress in Research on Nutrition and Cancer. New York: Wiley-Liss, 1990, pp. 135–143.

2. Rimer BK, Engstrom PF. Participation in macronutrient trials. In Micozzi M, Moon T (eds): Nutrition and Cancer Prevention: Investigating the Role of Macronutrients. New York: Marcel Dekker, in press.

3. Turk DC. Nonadherence to chemoprevention regimens: A ton of prevention. In Aiken LH, Mechanic D (eds): Applications of Social Sciences to Clinical Medicine and Health Policy. New Brunswick: Rutgers University Press, 1990, pp. 139–149.

4. Glanz K. Nutrition education for risk factor reduction and patient education: A review. Prev Med 14:721–752, 1985.

5. Arnold A, Johnstone B, Stoskopf B, Skingley P, Browman G, Levine M, Hryniuk W. Recruitment for an efficacy study in chemoprevention—The concerned smoker study. Prev Med 18:700–710, 1989.

6. Leventhal H, Nerenz DR, Leventhal EA, Love RR, Bendena LM. The behavioral dynamics of clinical trials. Presented at "Workshop: "Antiestrogen Prevention of Breast Cancer." Madison, WI, Oct 2–4, 1989.

7. Meichenbaum D, Turk DC (eds). Facilitating Treatment Adherence—A Practitioner's Guidebook. New York: Plenum Press, 1987.

8. Epstein LH, Cluss PA. A behavioral medicine perspective on adherence to long-term medical regimens. J Consult Clin Psychol 50:950–971, 1982.

9. Hansen WB, Collins LM, Malotte CK, Johnson CA, Fielding JE. Attrition in prevention research. J Behav Med 8(3):261–275, 1985.

10. Greenwald P, Sondik EJ, Young JL. Emerging roles for cancer registries in cancer control. Yale J Biol Med 59:561–566, 1986.

11. Zelen M. Are primary cancer prevention trials feasible? J Natl Cancer Inst 80(18):1442–1444, 1988.

12. Stevens M, Greenberg ER, Baron JA. Practical aspects of cancer prevention trials. In Moon T, Micozzi M (eds): Nutrition and Cancer Prevention. New York: Marcel Dekker, 1989, pp. 513–532.

13. Miller HH, Bauman LJ, DeCosse JJ. Psychosocial adjustment of familial polyposis patients and participation in a chemoprevention trial. Int J Psychiatry Med 16(3):211–230, 1986–87.

14. Gritz ER, DiMatteo MR, Hays RD. Methodological issues in adherence to cancer control regimens. Prev Med 18:711–720, 1989.

15. Powles TJ, Davey J, McKinna A. Chemoprevention of breast cancer. Acta Oncol 28:865–867, 1989.

16. Ho EE, Atwood JR, Meyskens FL Jr. Methodological development of dietary fiber intervention to lower colon cancer risk. In Engstrom PF, Mortenson LE, Anderson PN (eds): Advances in Cancer Control: The War on Cancer—15 Years of Progress. New York: Alan R. Liss, 1987, pp. 263–281.

17. Boyd NF, Cousins M, Beaton M, Fishell E, Wright B, Fish E, Kriukov V, Lockwood G, Tritchler D, Hanna W, Page DL. Clinical trial of low-fat, high-carbohydrate diet in subjects with mammographic dysplasia: Report of early outcomes. J Natl Cancer Inst 80(15):1244–1248, 1988.

18. Romney SL, Dwyer A, Slagle S, Duttagupta C, Palan PR, Basu J, Calderin S, Kadish A. Chemoprevention of cervix cancer: Phase I–II: A feasibility study involving the topical vaginal administration of retinyl acetate gel. Gynecol Oncol 20:109–119, 1985.

19. Steering Committee of the Physicians' Health Study Research Group. Final report on the aspirin component of the ongoing physicians' health study. N Engl J Med 321(3):129–135, 1989.

20. Dermatis H, Rowland J, Miransky J, Kerner J, Osborne M, Holland J. Consent and compliance in chemoprevention trials. In Proceedings: The First International Breast Cancer Chemoprevention Workshop. New York: Marcel Dekker, 1988, pp. 633–635.

21. Browman GP, Arnold A, Booker L, Johnstone B, Skingley P, Levine MN. Etretinate blood levels in monitoring of compliance and contamination in a chemoprevention trial. J Natl Cancer Inst 81:795–798, 1989.

22. Berenson M, Groshen S, Miller H, DeCosse J. Subject-reported compliance in a chemoprevention trial for familial adenomatous polyposis. J Behav Med 12(3):233–247, 1989.

23. Hong WK, Lippman SM, Itri LM, Karp DD, Lee JS, Byers RM, Schantz SP, Kramer AM, Lotan R, Peters LJ, Dimerly IW, Brown BW, Goepfert H. Prevention of second primary tumors with isotretinoin in squamous-cell carcinoma of the head and neck. N Engl J Med 323(12):795–801, 1990.

24. Henderson MM, Kushi LH, Thompson DJ, Gorbach SL, Clifford CK, Insull W, Moskowitz M, Thompson RS. Feasibility of a randomized trial of a low-fat diet for the prevention of breast cancer: Dietary compliance in the women's health trial vanguard study. Prev Med 19:115–133, 1990.

25. Morisky DE. Nonadherence to medical recommendations for hypertensive patients: Problems and potential solutions. Journal of Compliance in Health Care 1:5–20, 1986.

26. Becker MH, Maiman LA. Strategies for enhancing patient compliance. J Community Health 6:113–135, 1980.

27. Higbee M, Dukes G, Bosso J. Patient recall of physician's prescription instructions. Hospital Formulary 17:553–556, 1982.

28. Hays R, DiMatteo MR. Key issues and suggestions for patient compliance assessment. Journal of Compliance in Health Care 2:37–53, 1987.
29. Loescher LJ, Graham VE, Aickin M, Meyskens FL Jr, Surwit EA. Development of a contingency recruitment plan for a phase III chemoprevention trial of cervical dysplasia. Prog Clin Biol Res 339:151–163, 1990.
30. Chlebowski RT, Blackburn GL, Buzzard IM, Grosvenor M, Insull W, Nixon D, York RM, Khardekar J, Elashoff R, Wynder EL. Current status: Evaluation of dietary fat reduction as secondary breast cancer prevention. The Nutrition Adjuvant Study. In Aiken LH, Mechanic D (eds): Applications of Social Sciences to Clinical Medicine and Health Policy. New Brunswick, NJ: Rutgers University Press, 1986, 339:201–209.
31. Morris L, Halperin J. Effects of written drug information on patient knowledge and compliance: A literature review. Am J Public Health 69:47–52, 1979.
32. Ley P. Cognitive variables and noncompliance. Journal of Compliance in Health Care 1:171–188, 1986.
33. Turk DC, Salovey P, Litt MD. Adherence: A cognitive-behavioral perspective. In Gerber KE, Nehemkis AM (eds): Compliance: The Dilemma of the Chronically Ill. New York: Springer Publishing Company, 1986, pp. 44–72.
34. Black DM, Brand RJ, Greenlick M, Hughes G, Smith J. Compliance to treatment for hypertension in elderly patients: The SHEP pilot study. J Gerontol 42:552–557, 1987.
35. Cramer JA, Mattson RH, Prevey ML, Scheyer RD, Ouellette VL. How often is medication taken as prescribed? A novel assessment technique. JAMA 261:3273–3277, 1989.
36. Rimer BK, Trock B, Lerman C, King B, Engstrom PS. Why do some women get regular mammograms? Am J Prev Med (in press).
37. Bell RL, Curb JD, Friedman LM, McIntyre KM, Payton-Ross C, The BHAT Research Group. Enhancement of visit adherence in the national beta-blocker heart attack trial. Controlled Clin Trials 6:89–101, 1985.
38. Colletti G, Brownell K. The physical and emotional benefits of social support: Application to obesity, smoking, and alcoholism. In Hersen M, Eisler R, Miller PH (eds): Progress in Behavior Modification, vol. 13. New York: Academic Press, 1982, 109–178.
39. Agras WS, Bradford RH. Recruitment: An introduction. Circulation 66 (Suppl IV):2–5, 1982.
40. Marty PJ, McDermott RJ, Christiansen K. Evaluation of two pedagogical techniques for enhancing knowledge, attitudes and frequency of practice related to breast self-examination. Health Education, November/December:25–28, 1983.
41. Carmody TP. Promoting adherence to heart-healthy diets: A review of the literature. Journal of Compliance in Health Care 2(2):105–124, 1987.
42. Davis AL, Faust R, Ordenlich M. Self-help smoking cessation and maintenance programs: A comparative study with 12-month follow-up by the American Lung Association. Am J Public Health 74:1212–1217, 1984.
43. Glascow R, Schafer L, O'Neill HL. Self-help books and amount of therapist contact in smoking cessation programs. J Consult Clin Psychol 49:449–455, 1981.
44. Hoyt MF, Janis IL. Increasing adherence to a stressful decision via a motivational balance sheet procedure: A field experiment. J Pers Soc Psychol 31:833–839, 1975.
45. Prue DM, Davis CJ, Martin JE, Moss RA. An investigation of a minimal contact brand fading program for smoking treatment. Addict Behav 8:307–310, 1983.

A Population-based Trial of β-Carotene Chemoprevention of Head and Neck Cancer

Susan Taylor Mayne,[1] Tongzhang Zheng,[1] Dwight T. Janerich,[1]
W. Jarrard Goodwin, Jr.,[2] Barbara G. Fallon,[3]
Dennis L. Cooper,[4] and Craig D. Friedman[5]

[1]Cancer Prevention Research Unit for Connecticut at Yale
[4]Department of Medical Oncology
[5]Department of Surgery
Yale University School of Medicine
New Haven, Connecticut

[2]Department of Otolaryngology
University of Miami School of Medicine
Miami, Florida

[3]Section of Hematology/Oncology
St. Francis Hospital and Medical Center
Hartford, Connecticut

BACKGROUND

Squamous cell carcinoma (SCC) of the upper aerodigestive tract (oral cavity, pharynx, and larynx) is a major health problem in the United States and throughout the world. It is estimated that 43,300 new cases will be identified and that 11,800 patients will die of these cancers in the United States in 1991 (1). In addition to the number of patients affected, cancers of the oral cavity, pharynx, and larynx assume a higher relative importance because of the functional impairment and cosmetic deformity associated with the cancer and its treatment.

The incidence of oral cancers in women in Connecticut has been increasing (2,3), probably because of the increased level of tobacco exposure in females. Excluding cancer of the lip, the incidence of oral cancers in men in Connecticut has also been increasing (2). Without effective intervention, increased snuff and chewing tobacco use in children and young adults can also lead to a higher incidence of SCC of the oral cavity and pharynx in the future. Primary prevention, such as tobacco and alcohol cessation, is clearly the most desirable way to reduce risk in this population. However, tobacco and alcohol cessation programs have met with limited success, and those individuals who cease exposure may still be at increased risk (4). Another approach is needed as an adjunct to tobacco and alcohol cessation, and, to date, chemoprevention with inhibitory micronutrients is the most promising idea.

The Biology and Prevention of Aerodigestive Tract Cancers
Edited by G.R.Newell and W.K. Hong, Plenum Press, New York, 1992

119

With advances in early detection, approximately 50% of the patients now present early with Stage I or II disease. Although treatment given at this stage is relatively successful, failure remains all too common—mainly because of local recurrence and second primary cancers. Approximately 20% of Stage I or II patients have recurrence after definitive therapy with surgery or radiation, and 90% of these recurrences take place within the first 2 years (5). Second primary cancers, defined as those occurring a set distance from the initial primary cancer or more than 5 years later, are remarkably common in this group of patients. The expected incidence of second primary cancers varies, both by site (5–7) and by current tobacco habits (4,8); however, a reasonable estimate is that 4% of Stage I or II patients will develop second primary cancers yearly (or 20% over 5 years [9]). These second primary malignancies are divided approximately equally between the lungs, the esophagus, and the other upper aerodigestive tract sites (e.g., oral cavity, pharynx, and larynx [5,6,9]). The incidence and sites of second primary cancers have been described in the Connecticut population base, which we are studying (7).

The major risk factors for SCC of the upper aerodigestive tract are tobacco exposure and alcohol ingestion (10). In 90% of patients, diffuse, chronic exposure of the mucous membranes to these agents accounts for the common finding of "field cancerization" (11). This concept is central to understanding the cause of failure following localized treatment in patients who present with highly curable Stage I or II cancers.

Pharmacologic intervention (chemoprevention) could conceivably inhibit or reverse the development of these diffuse precancerous and cancerous changes in the epithelium. Ideally, a chemopreventive agent should be effective against tumor promotion/progression, nontoxic, easily administered, and relatively available and inexpensive. A variety of micronutrients are being examined as potential chemopreventive agents for various tumor sites (12). β-Carotene, a naturally occurring provitamin A compound, is essentially nontoxic and is readily available in foods and in synthetic form. More importantly, recent evidence suggests that β-carotene holds great potential for chemoprevention of cancer of the upper aerodigestive tract, as discussed below.

Epidemiologic Evidence

A growing body of evidence from epidemiologic studies suggests that dietary β-carotene may confer protection against certain types of cancer (see [13] for review). This association has most frequently been shown for lung cancer and, more specifically, SCC of the lung, although protection at a variety of other tumor sites has also been reported. For example, several recent case-control studies have reported that increased consumption of fruits and vegetables, the major dietary sources of β-carotene, is associated with reduced risk of oral cancer (14), oral and pharyngeal cancer (15), and laryngeal cancer (16,17). However, a population-based study of oral and pharyngeal cancers found a significant protective effect for carotene, vitamin C, and fiber from fruits, but not from vegetables (18).

Recognizing the inherent limitations of dietary assessment, some epidemiologic studies have examined the association between serum or plasma β-carotene levels and cancer risk. Ibrahim et al. (19) reported that plasma carotene levels were substantially lower in patients with cancer of the oral cavity or oropharynx than in matched controls (39.5 µg% vs. 61.5 µg%, respectively). Similar results were reported in a study of oral leukoplakia (20).

Animal Evidence

In concordance with the epidemiologic evidence, animal studies also support a role for β-carotene as a chemopreventive agent. Several animal studies have shown that the administration of β-carotene (topical, injected, or oral) inhibits carcinogenesis at a variety of tumor sites (13). Schwartz et al. have utilized the hamster buccal pouch model to demonstrate that β-carotene can inhibit and regress oral SCCs induced by dimethylbenz[*a*]anthracene (21–24). In a recent experiment, the mean oral tumor burden following β-carotene injection was 42.7 cu mm versus 2258.9 cu mm in the sham-injected control group (23). A possible mechanism for tumor regression is suggested by the finding that injection of β-carotene in the tumor-bearing site resulted in a dramatic increase in the number of macrophages staining positively for tumor necrosis factor (21). Protective effects were replicated when the animals were given oral versus injected β-carotene (22).

Clinical Evidence

Stich and co-workers have used the frequency of micronucleated cells in exfoliated oral mucosa to examine chemopreventive activity of β-carotene. These micronuclei, which mainly result from chromatid or chromosome fragments, are used to provide a marker for genotoxic damage in tissues from which oral carcinomas develop (25). Stich's group has consistently demonstrated that oral β-carotene supplementation (180 mg/wk) significantly decreases the frequency of micronucleated cells in buccal mucosa of high-risk populations (25–27). Another approach that has been used to examine potential chemopreventive agents for oral cancer is with leukoplakia, a precursor lesion for oral cancer. Garewal et al. (28) reported that β-carotene was an effective agent in treating oral leukoplakia and concluded that a lack of toxicity, coupled with strong indications of efficacy, make β-carotene a highly attractive chemopreventive agent for cancers of the oral cavity, pharynx, and larynx.

In summary, SCC of the upper aerodigestive tract is a significant clinical problem. The group at highest risk for developing these cancers is made up of those patients who have already been treated for their first primary tumor. Chemoprevention with β-carotene is an attractive possibility that has yet to be tested experimentally. Patients with all stages of disease may benefit from β-carotene administration, but patients with advanced disease are difficult to study because of high treatment-related morbidity and mortality, frequent intercurrent disease, and dysphagia (pill-taking is often difficult because of difficulty swallowing). Patients with Stage I or II disease are, as a group, more healthy, more highly motivated, and more likely to survive long enough to be at risk for the development of second primary malignancies. Thus, it seems timely and justified to conduct a clinical trial in patients with Stage I or II SCC of the upper aerodigestive tract to determine whether supplemental β-carotene is efficacious in reducing treatment failure.

STUDY DESIGN

This study is a randomized, double-blinded, and placebo-controlled trial whose primary objective is to determine whether supplemental β-carotene (50 mg/day) reduces the incidence of treatment failure owing to second primary tumors and local recurrences in patients treated curatively for early-stage cancers of the head and neck. A secondary objective of this trial is to establish that a high percentage of the individuals in this population will take and tolerate daily β-carotene supplements over a long period of time. An additional objective is to acquire prospective data on the relative frequency of second primary tumors and recurrences in patients with Stage I or II disease, depending upon age, site of the initial primary, treatment (radiation or surgery) of the initial primary cancer, nutritional status, and the presence or absence of continuing tobacco and alcohol exposures.

This trial is being conducted by the Cancer Prevention Research Unit (CPRU) for Connecticut at Yale University (New Haven, CT) and is population-based, with the study population consisting of all newly diagnosed cases of Stage I or II upper aerodigestive tract cancer in the state of Connecticut. While a multicenter design was considered an alternative approach for recruiting patients, such an approach would be problematic in this instance because of the larger research hospitals primarily treating referred cases of Stage III or IV cancer of the upper aerodigestive tract. In addition, a population-based recruitment strategy, as used in this study, has numerous other advantages. For example, the availability of a statewide tumor registry means that this trial can determine if patients who enroll in the trial have a similar failure and/or mortality experience to those who are not enrolled. Also, patients who are enrolled but subsequently lost to follow-up may be tracked for failure via the tumor registry. Finally, prior knowledge of 1) the number of patients available for study; 2) the names and specialties of their physicians; and 3) the hospital/geographic distribution of patients is a critical asset in trial planning.

Study Population

Recruitment for this trial began in December 1990, with the first patients being enrolled in January 1991. Newly diagnosed patients with upper aerodigestive tract cancer (including oral cavity, pharynx, and larynx) in Connecticut are ascertained via the Rapid Case Ascertainment (RCA) system established within the CPRU for Connecticut at Yale. In brief, the RCA system is an organized system in the state's 35 community hospitals that rapidly identifies essentially all incident cases of cancer in Connecticut. RCA staff have successfully guided this and other research protocols through each hospital's Institutional Review Board system. RCA staff then visit either the tumor registry or the pathology department at each hospital on a regular basis, to identify rapidly, newly diagnosed cases. The Connecticut Tumor Registry estimates that approximately 600 Connecticut residents are diagnosed with cancer of the oral cavity, pharynx, or larynx each year, with approximately 50% of them having either Stage I or II disease.

Once a potentially eligible patient has been identified, the patient is assigned to one of the clinical advisors to the study. The clinical advisor then contacts the patient's primary care physician by telephone (physician-to-physician contact) to assess patient eligibility and obtain physician consent to contact eligible patients. Patients are considered eligible for inclusion in the trial if they meet the following criteria: 1) recently diagnosed Stage I or Stage II SCC of the tongue (ICD #141), gum or mouth (ICD #143–145), oropharynx (ICD #146), hypopharynx (ICD #148), pharynx (ICD #149), or larynx (ICD #161). Patients with carcinoma in situ at the above-named sites are also eligible. Criteria for staging are those of the American Joint Committee for Cancer Staging and End Results Reporting; 2) resident of the state of Connecticut; 3) between 20 and 75 years of age; and 4) "disease free" at enrollment. In this instance, "disease free" means that the patient has completed treatment for the primary tumor and there is no evidence of residual cancer. A normal chest X ray is also required to aid in this determination. Patients are considered for inclusion only if they can be enrolled into the trial within 4 months of completing treatment.

Exclusion criteria are as follows: 1) Stage III or Stage IV carcinomas; 2) non-SCCs; 3) severe co-morbidities, some of which include AIDS, dementia, chemical evidence of significant hepatic dysfunction (total bilirubin > 1.8 mg%) or significant renal dysfunction (creatinine > 2.0 mg%), poorly compensated congestive heart failure, or severe malabsorption; 4) history of consuming supplemental retinol (>10,000 IU/day), carotene (>5 mg/day), α-tocopherol (>50 IU/day), selenium (>25 μg/day), or fish oil within the past year; 5) previous treatment for another upper aerodigestive tract cancer; and 6) synchronous primary tumor of the lung or esophagus.

Initial Contact/Consent

Eligible patients are sent a one-page introductory letter informing them of the purpose of the study and of their physician's approval. In addition, the letter states that a study nurse will be calling them to arrange a personal visit at their convenience. If the patient is willing, a study nurse then visits the patient in the patient's home or in the office of the patient's personal physician. The purpose of this initial visit is to establish personal contact with each patient (important for accrual and compliance); explain the purposes and requirements of the study and answer any questions the patient may have; obtain informed consent from those patients who agree to participate; complete an extensive baseline health history interview; obtain a venous blood sample; and provide a 1-month supply of capsules (placebo) to patients who agree to participate. The questionnaire includes sections on basic demographic information, medical history (including present illness), family health history, and risk factor history (specifically tobacco and alcohol exposures, dentition, and oral hygiene). The nurse also gives the patient a dietary questionnaire to complete during the next month.

This trial will utilize a 1-month placebo run-in period (29), which helps identify non-compliant patients or patients reporting considerable toxicity, so that they can be excluded from the trial before randomization. Longer run-in periods are often used in chemoprevention trials; however, a brief run-in period allows patients to begin their respective interventions more rapidly, which may be important regarding tumor recurrence. Patients are considered compliant if they consume more than 75% of the capsules that should have been consumed during this run-in period. If the patient is not compliant or decides to discontinue with the study, he or she is withdrawn from the study at this time.

INTERVENTION PROCEDURES

Randomization

A stratified randomization procedure will be employed in this clinical trial to ensure prognostic comparability between the two treatment groups. Stratification is on tumor site (oral cavity, pharynx, or larynx) and smoking history (<25 pack-years; ≥25 pack-years), because both are important prognostic factors (4,6–8,30). The randomization list was prepared as random permuted blocks, with a block size of 4 within each stratum and an allocation ratio of 1:1. The Yale Investigational Drug Service holds the randomization list and is responsible for treatment assignments.

Drug Formulation/Delivery

The intervention dose selected for this study is 50 mg of β-carotene daily per os. The dose of 50 mg of β-carotene per day was selected for the following reasons: 1) this population is at exceptionally high risk and, therefore, merits a dosage higher than that traditionally employed in chemoprevention trials with β-carotene (15–30 mg/day); 2) 50 mg of β-carotene has no greater toxicity than 15–30 mg of β-carotene, but may be more effective; and 3) 50 mg is the highest dose that can be formulated into a single capsule that is not so large as to make swallowing difficult. We had originally planned to administer the 50-mg β-carotene in combination with 5000 IU of retinol (as retinyl palmitate), but opted to delete retinol from the intervention for the following reasons: 1) recent reports from epidemiologic studies suggested that dietary levels of retinol could be positively associated with risk for oral and pharyngeal cancers (18) and esophageal cancers (31–34); 2) animal studies further suggested that retinol could potentiate upper aerodigestive tract cancers (35,36; Wargovich et al. [1991], unpublished data); 3) high levels of alcohol use, which are known to potentiate retinol toxicity (37), are observed in our population; 4) it is difficult to interpret the outcome of a combination intervention when a factorial design is not used. For example, if retinol increased but β-carotene reduced treatment failure, we would falsely conclude that β-carotene was ineffective as a chemopreventive agent in this clinical setting.

The β-carotene and placebo are obtained from BASF Corporation (Wyandotte, MI) and then encapsulated in opaque gelatin capsules. Capsules are packaged into calendar packs (Regional Service Center, Woburn, MA) and shipped to a drug repository (ERC Bioservices Corp., Rockville, MD). Short-term supplies of calendar packs are sent to the Yale/New Haven Hospital Pharmacy Investigational Drug Service, where the medication is catalogued, stored, and distributed to the nurse interviewers. The Investigational Drug Service also maintains a 24-hour telephone service in case of an emergency.

Study nurses will deliver the medication to the patients at the following time points: a 1-month supply at time –1 month (baseline, start of run-in), a 3-month supply at time 0 (randomization, post–run-in), and a 3-month supply at time 3 months. At 6 months, patients will be mailed a 6-month supply of capsules; at 12 months, the nurses will deliver the capsules to the patients, and then distribution (in person and via mail) will continue in 6-month increments for the duration of the trial.

Patient compliance to the treatments will be assessed as follows: capsules will be counted every 3 months initially and every 6 months thereafter; patients will be asked to record their capsule-taking behaviors on a calendar; and blood levels of β-carotene will be monitored as a crude indicator of compliance. The capsule count is considered the primary indicator of compliance. Methods to facilitate treatment adherence are currently being developed.

Clinical Follow-up

Because the end points for the study (tumor recurrence and second primary cancer) are readily identified with minimal diagnostic variability among physicians, patient follow-up for disease is done by the patient's regular physician. This manner of follow-up does not jeopardize the patient/physician relationship and presumably aids in accrual, as physicians are more likely to allow their patients to participate if follow-up is carried out as usual. Another advantage of having the patients' regular physicians do the follow-up is that it involves community physicians in cancer prevention efforts.

Physicians are asked to adhere to a uniform follow-up schedule, with the patient being seen at least every 6 weeks for the first year, every 3 months for the second and third years, and every 6 months for the fourth and fifth years. A baseline and yearly chest X ray are also required. This follow-up schedule is standard for patients with cancer of the upper aerodigestive tract. Physicians are sent periodic follow-up reports to be completed and returned in accordance with our recommended follow-up schedule.

The primary outcome measure to be examined in this trial is total failure, defined as either a local recurrence or a second primary tumor in the lung, esophagus, or another region of the upper aerodigestive tract. Another upper aerodigestive tract cancer is considered a second primary tumor only if it occurs more than 2 cm away from the site of the initial tumor in a patient treated by radiation, or more than 2 cm away from the suture line in a patient treated by surgery. One of our clinical advisors (W.J.G.) will review the data and make the final determination concerning recurrences versus second primary tumors. This decision will have no impact on the primary outcome measure of the study, which is total failure. In the event of a tumor recurrence or the occurrence of a second primary, we request that the physician send the appropriate slides to us for review. If it is lung cancer, we will also request the chest X-ray film for review. When either a second primary tumor occurs or there is local recurrence, the medication will be discontinued, and we will continue to follow the patient's outcome for the duration of the trial.

Assessment of Adverse Effects

We do not anticipate toxicity associated with the β-carotene supplement, because β-carotene is administered therapeutically for the treatment of erythropoietic protoporphyria at doses up to and exceeding 180 mg/day with no evidence of toxicity (38). Nonetheless, all subjects are asked to report any side effects at the end of the run-in and at the end of each 3-month interval. At a dose of 50 mg/day, it is expected that some of the subjects will experience carotenodermia, which is a harmless yellowing/tanning of the skin. All subjects are advised that this is a potential side effect associated with enrolling in this trial. The dose will be reduced to 50 mg every other day in patients who experience significant carotenodermia and are concerned about it for cosmetic reasons.

Biochemical Analyses

Blood is obtained by venipuncture and collected into 2×7.5-ml heparinized Vacutainer tubes (Beckton-Dickinson Co., Rutherford, NJ) at each nurse visit (−1 month, 0, 3, 12 months, and yearly thereafter) for the duration of the trial. Blood samples are protected from light and transported back to the laboratory in coolers. Plasma is aliquoted and stored at −70°C under nitrogen, pending analysis. Plasma β-carotene, retinol, and α-tocopherol are analyzed by reverse-phase high-performance liquid chromatography, according to established methods (39–41). (The plasma β-carotene analyses may be particularly valuable in identifying drop-ins [patients randomized to placebo who independently begin supplementing with β-carotene] and dropouts [patients randomized to β-carotene who terminate supplementation].) Plasma total cholesterol and total triglyceride are analyzed by Sigma Kit (Sigma Chemical Co., St. Louis, MO). To ensure quality control for the micronutrient analyses, this laboratory is participating in the National Institute of Standards and Technology's Micronutrient Measurement Proficiency Testing Program.

Dietary Analyses

Baseline and annual dietary information is collected by a questionnaire concerning the frequency of consumption of foods over the past year. This information is necessary because general nutritional status (undernutrition) has been reported to be a prognostic indicator in head and neck cancer (42). Such prospectively obtained dietary data (particularly on the placebo-supplemented group) may be valuable for future research studies concerning nutritional status and patient failure in this population.

Our questionnaire was developed by Dr. Gladys Block from the National Cancer Institute (43). It contains a list of 98 food items, representing at least 90% of the total U.S. caloric consumption, and is thought to be adequate for the assessment of a wide range of nutrients consumed in the typical U.S. diet. It also accounts for seasonality of intake, which may be particularly important in estimating β-carotene intake, because individuals will be enrolling in the trial throughout the year. We will also inquire about the use of vitamin and mineral supplements and alcohol.

Statistical Considerations

Because our interest is in improving the prognosis for these patients by extending the disease-free interval, the analysis will employ methods appropriate for failure-time data. To compute the number of patients we need to recruit, we used formulas appropriate for log-rank–type tests and proportional hazards models, assuming different lengths of accrual and follow-up (44,45). The calculations assume a two-sided, level 0.05 test, and 90% or 80% power, as specified. The baseline risk of failure owing to second primary tumors or recurrence within 5 years after "cure" was assumed to be 0.35. We arrived at this number by adding the incidence of local recurrence (20% over 5 years) to the incidence of second primary tumors (also approximately 20% over 5 years) and subtracting 5% because of the possibility of dual failure.

Based on these considerations, a sample size of 520 patients (260 per treatment group) would provide 90% power to detect a 40% reduction in the hazard rate, and 80% power to detect a 35% reduction in the hazard rate, if patients are accrued for 3.5 years and followed for an additional 4 years. We have thus set a target of enrolling 598 patients (520 + 15% to cover possible dropouts) who successfully complete the run-in period. These estimates require an accession rate of approximately 57% (598 of 1050 expected eligible patients), with a total project duration of 7.5 years plus additional time for analysis.

CONCLUSIONS

Patients who have been curatively treated for early-stage cancers of the upper aerodigestive tract are at exceptional risk of failure because of second malignant tumors and local recurrences. While numerous studies strongly suggest that β-carotene may be efficacious at inhibiting carcinogenesis of the upper aerodigestive tract, it must be emphasized that definitive evidence of a chemopreventive effect of β-carotene in humans is not available at this time. Consequently, the results of rigorously controlled clinical trials, such as the one described in this report, are critically needed and eagerly anticipated.

ACKNOWLEDGMENT

This research is supported by a National Institutes of Health grant CA-42101.

REFERENCES

1. Boring C, Squires TS, Tong T. Cancer Statistics 1991. CA: A Cancer Journal for Clinicians 41:19–31, 1991.
2. Chen J, Katz RV, Krutchkoff DJ. Intraoral squamous cell carcinoma: Epidemiologic patterns in Connecticut from 1935 to 1985. Cancer 66:1288–1296, 1990.
3. Chen J, Katz RV, Krutchkoff DJ. Epidemiology of oral cancer in Connecticut, 1935 to 1985. Cancer 65:2796–2802, 1990.
4. Wynder EL, Dodo H, Bloch DA, Gantt RC, Moore OS. Epidemiologic investigation of multiple primary cancer of the upper alimentary and respiratory tracts: I. A retrospective study. Cancer 24:730–739, 1969.
5. Jesse RH, Fletcher GH, Lindberg RD, Daly TE, Matalon V, Luna MA. Cancer of the head and neck. In Clark RL, Howe CD (eds): Cancer Patient Care at M. D. Anderson Hospital and Tumor Institute. Chicago: Year Book Medical Publishers, 1976, pp. 89–124.
6. Wagenfield DH, Harwood AR, Bryce DP. Second primary respiratory tract malignancies in glottic carcinoma. Cancer 46:1883–1886, 1980.
7. Winn DM, Blot WJ. Second cancer following cancers of the buccal cavity and pharynx in Connecticut. NCI Monogr 68:25–48, 1985.
8. Moore C. Cigarette smoking and cancer of the mouth, pharynx and larynx: A continuing study. JAMA 218:553–558, 1971.
9. Odette J, Szymanowski RT, Nichols RD. Multiple head and neck malignancies. Transactions of the American Academy of Ophthalmologists and Otolaryngologists 84:805–813, 1977.
10. Rothman KJ. Epidemiology of head and neck cancer. Laryngoscope 88:435–438, 1978.
11. Slaughter DP, Southwick HW, Smejkal W. "Field cancerization" in oral stratified squamous epithelium. Cancer 5:963–968, 1953.
12. Bertram JS, Kolonel LK, Meyskens FL, Jr. Rationale and strategies for chemoprevention of cancer in humans. Cancer Res 47:3012–3031, 1987.
13. Mayne ST. Beta-carotene and cancer prevention: What is the evidence? Conn Med 54:547–551, 1990.
14. Zheng T, Boyle P, Willett WC, Hu HF, Duan J, Evstifeeva T, Niu S, MacMahon B. Nutritional factors, dietary practices and risk of oral cancer: A case control study in Beijing, People's Republic of China. Int J Cancer, in press.
15. Winn DM, Ziegler RG, Pickle LW, Gridley G, Blot WJ, Hoover RN. Diet in the etiology of oral and pharyngeal cancer among women from the southern United States. Cancer Res 44:1216–1222, 1984.
16. De Stefani D, Correa P, Oreggia F, Leiva J, Rivero S, Fernandez G, Deneo-Pellegrini H, Zavala D, Fontham E. Risk factors for laryngeal cancer. Cancer 60:3087–3091, 1987.
17. La Vecchia C, Negri E, D'Avanzo B, Franceschi S, Decarli A, Boyle P. Dietary indicators of laryngeal cancer risk. Cancer Res 50:4497–4500, 1990.

18. McLaughlin JK, Gridley G, Block G, Winn DM, Preston-Martin S, Schoenberg JB, Greenberg RS, Stemhagen A, Austin DF, Ershow AG, Blot WJ, Fraumeni JF. Dietary factors in oral and pharyngeal cancer. J Natl Cancer Inst 80:1237–1243, 1988.
19. Ibrahim K, Jafarey NA, Zuberi SJ. Plasma vitamin A and carotene levels in squamous cell carcinoma of oral cavity and oropharynx. Clin Oncol 3:203–207, 1977.
20. Wahi PN, Podhke RR, Arora S, Sriustaua MD. Serum vitamin A studies in leukoplakia and carcinoma of the oral cavity. Indian Journal of Pathology and Bacteriology 5:10–16, 1962.
21. Schwartz J, Suda D, Light G. Beta-carotene is associated with the regression of hamster buccal pouch carcinoma and the induction of tumor necrosis factor in macrophages. Biochem Biophys Res Commun 136:1130–1135, 1986.
22. Schwartz J, Sloane D, Shklar G. Immune surveillance enhancement associated with carotenoid inhibition of oral cancer in hamster buccal pouch model. Presented at the 8th International Symposium on Carotenoids, 1987, Boston, MA, Abstract 50.
23. Schwartz J, Shklar G. Regression of experimental oral carcinomas by local injection of beta-carotene and canthaxanthin. Nutr Cancer 11:35–40, 1988.
24. Suda D, Schwartz J, Shklar G. Inhibition of experimental oral carcinogenesis by topical beta-carotene. Carcinogenesis 7:711–715, 1986.
25. Stich HF, Stich W, Rosin MP, Vallejera MO. Use of the micronucleus test to monitor the effect of vitamin A, beta-carotene and canthaxanthin on the buccal mucosa of betel nut/tobacco chewers. Int J Cancer 34:745–750, 1984.
26. Stich HF, Hornby AP, Dunn BP. A pilot beta-carotene intervention trial with Inuits using smokeless tobacco. Int J Cancer 36:321–327, 1985.
27. Stich HF, Rosin MP, Hornby AP, Mathew B, Sankaranarayanan R, Nair MK. Human intervention studies with carotenoids. Presented at the 8th International Symposium on Carotenoids, 1987, Boston, MA, Abstract 45.
28. Garewal H, Meyskens FL, Jr, Killen D, Reeves D, Kiersch TA, Elletson H, Strosberg A, King D, Steinbronn K. Response of oral leukoplakia to beta-carotene. J Clin Oncol 8:1715–1720, 1990.
29. Hennekens CH. Issues in the design and conduct of clinical trials. J Natl Cancer Inst 73:1473–1476, 1984.
30. Jesse RH, Sugarbaker EV. Carcinoma of the oropharynx: Why we fail. Am J Surg 132:435–438, 1976.
31. Tuyns AJ, Riboli LE, Doornbos G, Pequignot G. Diet and esophageal cancer in Calvados (France). Nutr Cancer 9:81–92, 1987.
32. Brown LM, Blot WJ, Schuman SH, Smith VM, Ershow AG, Marks RD, Fraumeni JF, Jr. Environmental factors and high risk of esophageal cancer among men in coastal South Carolina. J Natl Cancer Inst 80:1620–1625, 1988.
33. Decarli A, Liati P, Negri E, Franceschi S, La Vecchia C. Vitamin A and other dietary factors in the etiology of esophageal cancer. Nutr Cancer 10:29–37, 1987.
34. Graham S, Marshall J, Haughey B, Brasure J, Freudenheim J, Zielezny M, Wilkinson G, Nolan J. Nutritional epidemiology of cancer of the esophagus. Am J Epidemiol 131:454–467, 1990.
35. Levij IS, Polliack A. Potentiating effect of vitamin A on 9-10 dimethyl,1-2 benzanthracene-carcinogenesis in the hamster cheek pouch. Cancer 22:300–306, 1968.
36. Levij IS, Polliack A. Lymphoma-like lesions induced in the hamster cheek pouch with topical vitamin A palmitate. Pathol Microbiol 34:282–288, 1969.
37. Hathcock JN, Hattan DG, Jenkins MY, McDonald JT, Sundaresan PR, Wilkening VL. Evaluation of vitamin A toxicity. Am J Clin Nutr 52:183–202, 1990.
38. Mathews-Roth MM. Photosensitization by porphyrins and prevention of photosensitization by carotenoids. J Natl Cancer Inst 69:279–285, 1982.
39. Bieri JG, Brown ED, Smith JC, Jr. Determination of individual carotenoids in human plasma by high performance liquid chromatography. Journal of Liquid Chromatography 8:473–484, 1985.
40. Ruddat M, Will OH. High-performance liquid chromatography of carotenoids. Methods Enzymol 111:189–200, 1985.
41. Catignani GL. An HPLC method for the simultaneous determination of retinol and alpha-tocopherol in plasma or serum. Methods Enzymol 123:215–219, 1986.
42. Brookes GB. Nutritional status: A prognostic indicator in head and neck cancer. Otolaryngol Head Neck Surg 93:69–74, 1985.
43. Block G, Hartman AM, Dresser CM, Carroll MD, Gannon J, Gardner L. A data-based approach to diet questionnaire design and testing. Am J Epidemiol 124:453–469, 1986.
44. Schoenfeld DA, Richter JR. Nomograms for calculating the number of patients needed for a clinical trial with survival as an endpoint. Biometrics 38:163–170, 1982.
45. Schoenfeld DA. Sample-size formulas for the proportional hazards regression model. Biometrics 39:499–503, 1983.

Chemoprevention of Barrett's Esophagus and Oral Leukoplakia

Harinder S. Garewal

Cancer Prevention and Control
University of Arizona Cancer Center
Department of Veterans Affairs Medical Center
Tucson, Arizona

Studies of premalignant lesions constitute an important approach to devising strategies for preventing cancer. Cancer develops through a series of sequential steps involving initiation, promotion, and progression to invasive malignancy. However, many of the early steps in this pathway are reflected as changes at the subcellular level only and, therefore, cannot be identified phenotypically as clinical lesions. Premalignant lesions are often the first clinically recognizable lesions that can be used to identify a tissue affected by carcinogens. Barrett's esophagus and oral leukoplakia, for example, are considered premalignant lesions for esophageal adenocarcinoma and oral cancer, respectively. Lesions such as these characterize one of the better-defined, intermediate end points whose reversal or suppression can be studied to evaluate useful approaches for the overall chemoprevention of cancer.

BARRETT'S ESOPHAGUS

Barrett's esophagus is a condition in which the esophageal mucosa is lined by metaplastic columnar epithelium rather than by normal, stratified squamous epithelium (1,2). The major contributing factor to its etiology is chronic gastroesophageal reflux. However, neither the cell nor the tissue of origin of the abnormal epithelium has been definitively identified.

Barrett's esophagus is not an uncommon lesion. Recent studies have shown that as many as 12% of all patients with reflux symptoms (e.g., heartburn) who are evaluated by endoscopy and biopsy, will have Barrett's esophagus (3). Furthermore, a majority of cases of Barrett's esophagus remain unrecognized, with recent comparisons between clinically diagnosed Barrett's antemortem and autopsy prevalence suggesting that perhaps only one in 20 cases is recognized prior to death (4).

One of the most serious complications of Barrett's esophagus is its malignant potential (i.e., an increased risk of adenocarcinoma of the esophagus). Prevalence studies suggest an 8–40% occurrence of cancer in this lesion (2,5). Incidence studies, which are primarily retrospective, suggest a 30–40-fold increase in esophageal cancer risk in this population compared with the general population (6). Hence, the lesion is considered premalignant, and regular endoscopic surveillance and histologic examination are recommended for patients with Barrett's esophagus.

The Biology and Prevention of Aerodigestive Tract Cancers
Edited by G.R.Newell and W.K. Hong, Plenum Press, New York, 1992

We are studying Barrett's esophagus as a model premalignant lesion for adenocarcinoma because it has several unique characteristics. First, it represents a type of epithelium not normally present in the esophagus. Therefore, it is easier to identify the abnormal tissue that leads to adenocarcinoma than to the usual squamous cell esophageal cancers. Interestingly, adenocarcinoma of the esophagus has been reported with increasing frequency in recent studies (2). Second, Barrett's esophagus can be repeatedly accessed by modern fiberoptic endoscopic techniques. Furthermore, once the lesion appears in a patient, spontaneous regression or disappearance is extremely rare. Therefore, the natural history of Barrett's esophagus within one patient can be studied by serial longitudinal evaluations. In contrast, other premalignant lesions, such as colonic polyps, are usually removed after they are identified. Finally, Barrett's esophagus is a model for premalignant metaplasia. Metaplasia (i.e., the replacement of one adult tissue type by another) undoubtedly occurs as a premalignant change preceding many cancers, such as lung cancer. However, there are no other good models for premalignant metaplasia that are easily quantifiable and suitable for longitudinal follow-up.

In our studies, we have concentrated on areas of potential clinical usefulness. These include laboratory studies of biologic characteristics that might be useful as intermediate markers of cancer risk and clinical intervention trials using potential chemopreventive agents (Table 1).

Laboratory Studies

One intermediate marker is ornithine decarboxylase (ODC), the first enzyme in poly-amine biosynthesis (7). Its induction is thought to be important in carcinogenesis (8). ODC activity is altered in certain premalignant human conditions, such as familial polyposis of the colon (9), and is greater in adenomatous polyps than in normal colon mucosa (10–12). We compared ODC activity in endoscopic biopsies of Barrett's mucosa with normal upper gastrointestinal mucosa from the same patient derived from squamous esophagus, stomach, and small bowel. ODC activity was significantly greater in Barrett's mucosa than in the other tissues (13–15). Furthermore, in a small cohort of patients, ODC activity in Barrett's mucosa was greater in the presence of dysplasia than in its absence (14). Since polyamines are the effector molecules in this pathway, we quantitated polyamine content in Barrett's mucosal biopsies to correlate them with the increased ODC activity. Interestingly, there was no relationship between individual polyamine levels or between total polyamine content and the ODC activity (15). This intriguing finding suggests that the regulation of the polyamine pathway may be different in this premalignant tissue than in normal cells.

Recently, attempts have been made to correlate flow cytometric analyses of DNA content, another possible intermediate marker, with the presence of dysplasia and carcinoma in Barrett's esophagus (16–18). We have analyzed 169 biopsies obtained from 39 patients and documented that dysplasia can occur in the absence of flow cytometric abnormalities and, conversely, that the latter can be present in the absence of dysplasia. Reports by other investigators agree with these results (19). This observation raises the possibility that flow cytometric abnormalities may be a determinant of cancer risk independent of dysplasia or may precede the development of histologic changes. The long-term goal of this study is to assess whether cancer risk in Barrett's esophagus is limited to patients with dysplasia or aneuploidy, or both. If the increased cancer risk associated with Barrett's esophagus is confined to patients

Table 1. Studies in Barrett's Esophagus

- Ornithine decarboxylase and the polyamine pathway
- Flow cytometric abnormalities
- Tissue culture and use of cultured cells for cytogenetics and screening of potential chemopreventive agents
- Clinical intervention trials (13-*cis*–retinoic acid; α-DFMO)

with flow cytometric abnormalities (or dysplasia, or both), then the obvious clinical advantage would be the limitation of surveillance to such subjects only. The majority of patients belong in the "no dysplasia, no flow cytometric abnormality" category. If this group indeed has little or no increase in cancer risk compared with the normal population, it might be possible to decrease or even discontinue surveillance endoscopies, thereby saving a significant amount of medical care costs.

We have also developed a procedure for culturing epithelial cells from endoscopic biopsies of Barrett's mucosa (20). Early passages of these cultures have been used for karyotypic analysis, and clonal cytogenetic abnormalities have been identified (21). Clinical follow-up of these patients is continuing in order to determine whether the presence of karyotypic abnormalities will correlate with the incidence of malignancy. The cultured cells have been used to study the effect of potential chemopreventive agents on growth inhibition (22). Agents tested thus far include retinoids (13-*cis*–retinoic acid and 4-hydroxyphenyl-retinamide), carotenoids (β-carotene and canthaxanthin), and the ODC inhibitor α-difluoro-methylornithine (α-DFMO). Whereas the retinoids and carotenoids did not significantly inhibit the growth of the cultured cells, α-DFMO did.

Clinical Intervention Trials

Clinical intervention trials to assess chemoprevention possibilities were begun at the same time that the laboratory studies were initiated. At present, there is no standard treatment for Barrett's esophagus which does not reverse itself, even with aggressive medical or surgical antireflux therapy.

Our first study, with 13-*cis*–retinoic acid at a dose of 1 mg/kg/day, was based on this agent's activity in other premalignant lesions, such as oral leukoplakia. As expected, considerable toxicity was noted at this dose, and only 11 of 16 patients completed at least 6 weeks of treatment. No response was noted in these 11 patients, either in extent or in histology of the lesion (23). In addition to the usual toxicities associated with this drug, esophageal ulcers developed in the Barrett's mucosa of two patients. These healed on discontinuation of the treatment (24). The lack of efficacy of this agent may have been due to the short duration of the study, but, as emphasized above, toxicity prohibited a longer trial.

The next trial was with α-DFMO at a low dose of 0.5 g/m^2 t.i.d. Although α-DFMO has considerable toxicity when used at its maximum dose of about 4–6 g/m^2/day (i.e., the dose employed in trials for advanced malignancy), our objective was to test whether a low dose of α-DFMO, potentially useable in chemoprevention studies, would result in measurable changes in polyamine content in upper GI mucosa. Eight patients were treated for 6 weeks with α-DFMO. Polyamine content was measured at the beginning and completion of the treatment. Statistically significant changes in polyamine content were noted (approximately a 60% decrease in the spermidine-to-spermine ratio, primarily from a decrease in spermidine content). These changes occurred in the Barrett's mucosa as well as in normal tissue from squamous esophagus, gastric, and small-bowel mucosa. This was the first demonstration that a low dose of α-DFMO could produce significant changes in the polyamine pathway in human GI mucosa. Additional trials of potential chemopreventive agents are planned, either alone or in combination with antireflux agents.

ORAL LEUKOPLAKIA

Oral leukoplakia is a white patch or plaque on the mucosa that cannot be rubbed off and is not attributable to another specific disease entity. In general, it has a rather low malignant potential, probably less than 1% per year (25). When erythroplakia, a reddish component of the lesion, or severe dysplasia is present, the risk of cancer increases considerably. Oral and pharyngeal cancers together constitute the sixth most common cancers in the world in both sexes (26). Their incidence varies from region to region and in some developing countries, up to 25% of all cancers are found in the mouth (27,28). This variation in incidence has been related to known etiologic agents, the most important of which are tobacco and alcohol. Tobacco, either smoked or chewed, causes over 70% of oral cancers (29). Multiple cancers in the same patient are not infrequent and can occur either synchronously or metachronously with the primary tumor. Based on observations of the increased incidence of multiple tumors and precancerous changes of the aerodigestive tract in patients with oral cancer, the important theory of "field cancerization" was proposed. Essentially, this term refers to diffuse mucosal changes, presumably resulting from carcinogen exposure, that lead to cancer formation at multiple sites.

Recent evidence suggests a role for nutritional agents in the inhibition of oral carcinogenesis, particularly those related to vitamin A (the retinoids and carotenoids). In fact, recent intervention trials with these compounds in people at risk for oral cancer have produced results that show promising potential for cancer chemoprevention.

Epidemiologic and biologic evidence of a role for these agents has been the subject of several recent reviews (30). Moreover, experiments using animal models have shown a marked inhibitory effect on oral carcinogenesis, particularly in the hamster cheek pouch model system (31–33).

In human clinical trials, mucosa that has undergone field cancerization can be recognized in several ways. First, the abnormal expression of intermediate markers may be demonstrable. In this context, the only marker that has been the subject of clinical intervention trials is micronuclei formation. Micronucleated oral mucosal cells have been reported to be increased in people at risk for oral cancer, particularly in India and Southeast Asia, where betel nut, tobacco, and lime chewing are prevalent (34). Orally administered β-carotene and vitamin A decreased the number of micronuclei. A second way to identify affected mucosa is to study subjects who have been cured of early-stage oral cancer. These patients are at increased risk for developing a second primary tumor (35–37), hence, the implication that their mucosa has undergone field cancerization. (This topic is the subject of another paper in these proceedings.) Finally, the presence of premalignant lesions, leukoplakia or erythroplakia, can be used to identify affected mucosa. Several clinical trials have demonstrated the ability of retinoids and carotenoids to produce improvement in these premalignant lesions. In this paper, we focus on the leukoplakia trials.

The ultimate objectives of chemoprevention trials using subjects with leukoplakia are important when designing such studies. If the objective is to develop a treatment applicable to a small minority of patients with erythroplakia, high-grade dysplasia, or both whose conditions are not amenable to standard treatments such as reduction in local irritants, surgical excision, or cryosurgery, then some degree of toxicity in the treatment may be acceptable. Included in this category would be the use of active agents such as topical bleomycin and 5-fluorouracil (38). However, if the objective is the chemoprevention of cancer, with leukoplakia as a lesion in which to judge the activity of potential agents, then toxic agents are unlikely to be of practical benefit, even if they are effective.

Several trials have now shown that various retinoids, both natural and synthetic, can reverse leukoplakia. The efficacy of high doses of vitamin A in reversing the hyperkeratosis associated with leukoplakia has been known for over 25 years. However, until synthetic retinoids became available, the toxicity associated with high-dose vitamin A precluded further intervention trials. In earlier studies, Koch showed that 13-*cis*–retinoic acid, *trans*-retinoic acid, and etretinate each could produce objective responses in 60–90% of patients (39). Nevertheless, these drugs also resulted in considerable toxicity, particularly mucocutaneous, and relapses were frequent after therapy was discontinued.

More recent trials with retinoids and carotenoids are summarized in Table 2. In a randomized trial of 13-*cis*–retinoic acid, Hong et al. reported a response rate of 67% in 24

Table 2. Results of Recent Retinoid/Carotenoid Trials in Leukoplakia

Agent	CR (%)	PR (%)	OR (%)	Investigator
13-*cis*–retinoic acid	8	59	67	Hong et al. (40)
β-carotene	15	ND	ND	Stich et al. (34)
β-carotene + vitamin A	27	ND	ND	Stich et al. (34)
Vitamin A	57	ND	ND	Stich et al. (41)
β-carotene	8	63	71	Garewal et al. (42)

Abbreviations: CR, complete response; PR, partial response; OR, overall response; ND, not determined.

treated patients (40). The dose used, 1–2 mg/kg/day, was also toxic. Once again, relapses were frequent after treatment was discontinued, and some appeared to occur even while the treatment was being given (i.e., during the 3-month treatment period of the study) (see Figure 2 in ref. [40]).

Stich and colleagues performed several trials in India using vitamin A alone or in combination with β-carotene (34,41). Their studies differed from the other trials in that the lesions in the Indian patients were primarily related to the chewing of betel nut, mixed with other substances, and the population studied probably suffered from vitamin A deficiency. In one trial, Group I was given 180 mg/week of β-carotene, Group II was given β-carotene plus 100,000 IU/week of vitamin A, and Group III was given a placebo for 6 months (34). Approximately 15% of the patients in Group I and 27.5% in Group II had *complete* remissions of their disease, compared with 3% in Group III. In a more recent trial using a high dose of vitamin A alone, 200,000 IU/week for 6 months, the same group of investigators reported a 57% *complete* response rate, with the total suppression of new lesions (41).

In a pilot study conducted by our group, a response rate of 71% was observed in 24 patients who were given β-carotene alone at a dose of 30 mg/day (42). In this study and those mentioned above, relapses were very frequent, suggesting that continued maintenance treatment may be necessary to continue suppression of these lesions.

In interpreting the above studies and developing a strategy for the prevention of oral cancer, several issues should be kept in perspective. These are discussed briefly below:

1. Clinical response criteria: It is often difficult to apply standard "oncologic" definitions of response to oral leukoplakia. This is because leukoplakia is a lesion that can be directly visualized. Hence, marked improvement and thinning of the lesion are often apparent on visual examination but are difficult to quantitate in a manner similar to that used in therapeutic trials of anticancer agents. In the latter, the responding lesion is often visualized and measured on a radiograph or some other scan. Therefore, although investigators attempt to define a response by applying the standard 50% reduction in the product of the two longest diameters of lesions, doing so with any degree of precision is by no means easy when evaluating leukoplakia. Obviously, one approach would be to consider only complete responses, as Stich et al. have done (33,41). However, one would risk discarding potentially valuable modalities in short duration trials since, even though quantitating them is difficult, many lesions improve dramatically, and this may signify considerable activity of the agent being tested.

2. Role of histologic evaluation: Interpreting so-called histologic responses deserves considerable scrutiny. Dysplasia and other histologic abnormalities are not uniformly distributed throughout a premalignant or other lesion, including those occurring in the oral cavity. In other precancerous conditions, such as ulcerative colitis, Barrett's esophagus, esophageal dysplasia, and cervical dysplasia, the distribution of dysplasia is patchy with respect to its presence or absence and to degree (43,44). In addition, there is considerable intra- and interobserver variability in quantitating the degree of such change in an individual biopsy (43). Therefore, comparing only two biopsies, often taken weeks to months apart, to quantitate the degree of dysplasia is an approach subject to serious error. This is not to say that histologic follow-up is of no use at all. Its greatest usefulness lies in the setting of complete clinical responses, where it would be important to show that epithelial maturation is also normalized at the histologic level. Cases showing partial or no clinical response to treatment that are alleged to have improved histologically in degree of dysplasia may be acceptable as response criteria if this improvement is demonstrated in a series of follow-up biopsies that show little to no "oscillations" of dysplasia grade from one biopsy to another. Otherwise, changes from a single pretreatment biopsy to a single follow-up posttreatment biopsy will probably reflect sampling and interpretation errors rather than a true change in grade of dysplasia. Recognizing these difficulties with quantitating changes in hyperplasia and dysplasia, Stich et al. have attempted to develop other histologic and cytologic criteria (41). These, too, must be validated before they can be accepted as response criteria on their own.

Given these limitations, our approach has been to evaluate clinical and histologic changes together before arriving at a response designation.

3. Toxicity of agents: "Acceptable" toxicity of an agent clearly depends on the eventual use of the agent. Potential chemopreventive agents for the primary "prevention" of cancer must be essentially nontoxic to allow widespread use. Availability of a chemopreventive agent as a nutrient is advantageous since the agent can then be supplemented by dietary adjustments. Also, cost should not be completely prohibitive in developing countries, some of which face serious problems with oral cancer.

Considering the toxicity issues mentioned above, it is evident that toxic agents such as bleomycin, 13-*cis*–retinoic acid, and *trans*-retinoic acid are not suitable for use in the large-scale prevention of primary oral cancer, even if they are active. Large populations would need to be treated, and close toxicity monitoring is not feasible. Thus, further study is needed of essentially nontoxic agents such as β-carotene, low doses of vitamin A (<25,000 IU/day), and vitamin E (which is active in animal models but not yet tested clinically). In other situations, such as prevention of second primary tumors, where the cancer risk may be high enough to justify some toxicity, the use of other agents, such as low-dose 13-*cis*–retinoic acid, may be justifiable.

In summary, retinoids and carotenoids have shown their ability to reverse oral leukoplakia in recent trials of short duration. Additional, longer controlled trials with these agents are now under way. Depending on their results, strategies will need to be devised for using these agents in populations at risk to actually prevent oral cancer, whether as the primary tumor or a second cancer.

ACKNOWLEDGMENTS

Supported, in part, by National Cancer Institute grant 25702.

The invaluable assistance and collaboration of colleagues and co-workers are gratefully acknowledged. Particular thanks to the following: Richard E. Sampliner, MD; Brian Fennerty, MD; E. Gerner, PhD; and F. Meyskens, MD.

REFERENCES

1. Barrett NR. Chronic peptic ulcer of the esophagus and "esophagitis." Br J Surg 38:178–182, 1950.
2. Sjogren RW, Johnson LF. Barrett's esophagus: A review. Am J Med 74:313–321, 1983.
3. Winters C, Spurling TJ, Chobanian SJ, Curtis DJ, Esposito RL, Hacker JF, Johnson DA, Cruess DF, Cotelingam JD, Gurney MS, Cattau EL. Barrett's esophagus: A prevalent occult complication of gastroesophageal reflux disease. Gastroenterology 92:118–124, 1987.
4. Cameron EL, Zinsmeister ER, Ballard DJ, Carney JE. Prevalence of columnar-lined (Barrett's) esophagus: Comparison of population-based clinical and autopsy findings. Gastroenterology 99:918–922, 1990.

5. Naef AP, Savary M, Ozzello L. Columnar-lined lower esophagus: An acquired lesion with malignant predisposition. Report on 140 cases of Barrett's esophagus with 12 adenocarcinomas. J Thorac Cardiovasc Surg 70:826–835, 1975.

6. Cameron AJ, Ott BJ, Payne WP. The incidence of adenocarcinoma in columnar-lined (Barrett's) esophagus. N Engl J Med 313:857–859, 1985.

7. Pegg AE, McCann PP. Polyamine metabolism and function. Am J Physiol 243:C212–C221, 1982.

8. Verma AK, Boutwell RK. Inhibition of carcinogenesis by inhibitors of putrescine biosynthesis. In McCann PP, Pegg AE, Sjoerdsma A (eds): Inhibition of Polyamine Metabolism. Orlando, FL: Academic Press, 1987, pp. 249–258.

9. Luk GD, Baylin SB. ODC as a biologic marker in familial colonic polyposis. N Engl J Med 311:80–83, 1984.

10. Rozhin J, Wilson PS, Bull AW, Nigro ND. Ornithine decarboxylase activity in the rat and human colon. Cancer Res 44:3326–3330, 1984.

11. Lamurglia GM, Lacaine F, Malt RA. High ornithine decarboxylase activity and polyamine levels in human colorectal neoplasia. Ann Surg 204:89–93, 1986.

12. Sloan D, Garewal HS, Hixson L, Sampliner RE, Fennerty MB. ODC activity in colonic neoplasms. Proceedings of the American Association for Cancer Research, in press.

13. Garewal HS, Sampliner R, Kogan F, Smith W, Gerner E, Alberts D, Kendall D. Ornithine decarboxylase levels in Barrett's esophagus: A premalignant lesion for adenocarcinoma. Proceedings of the American Society of Clinical Oncology 5:18, 1986.

14. Garewal HS, Sampliner R, Gerner E, Steinbronn K, Alberts D, Kendall D. Ornithine decarboxylase activity in Barrett's esophagus: A potential marker for dysplasia. Gastroenterology 94:819–821, 1988.

15. Garewal HS, Gerner EW, Sampliner R, Roe D. Ornithine decarboxylase and polyamine levels in columnar upper gastrointestinal mucosae in patients at risk for adenocarcinoma. Cancer Res 48:3288–3291, 1988.

16. Garewal HS, Sampliner RE, Fennerty MB. Flow cytometry in Barrett's esophagus. What have we learned so far? Dig Dis Sci, in press.

17. Reid BF, Haggitt RC, Rubin CE, Rabinovitch PS. Barrett's esophagus: Correlation between flow cytometry and histology in detection of patients at risk for adenocarcinoma. Gastroenterology 93:1–11, 1987.

18. Fennerty MB, Way D, Sampliner R, Riddell R, Sloan D, Garewal HS. Discordance between flow cytometry and dysplasia in patients with Barrett's esophagus. Gastroenterology 94:A143, 1988.

19. McKinley MK, Budman DR, Grueneberg D, Bronzo RL, Weissman GS, Kahn E. DNA content in Barrett's esophagus and esophageal malignancy. Am J Gastroenterol 82:1012–1015, 1987.

20. Garewal HS, Leibovitz A, Sampliner R, Prabhala R, Trent J, Korc M, Sloan D. Tissue culture and characterization of epithelial cells derived from Barrett's esophagus: A premalignant lesion. Gastroenterology 94:A143, 1988.

21. Garewal HS, Sampliner RE, Liu Y, Trent JM. Chromosomal rearrangements in Barrett's esophagus, a premalignant lesion of esophageal adenocarcinoma. Cancer Genet Cytogenet 42:281–296, 1989.

22. Garewal HS, Prabhala R, Sampliner R, Sloan D. Effect of potential differentiating agents on the growth of Barrett's esophagus-derived epithelial cell cultures. Clin Res 36:131A, 1988.

23. Sampliner RE, Garewal HS. Phase II trial of 13-*cis* retinoic acid (isotretinoin) in Barrett's esophagus. Gastroenterology 94:A396, 1988.

24. Fennerty MB, Sampliner RE, Garewal HS. Esophageal ulceration associated with 13-cis-retinoic acid therapy in patients with Barrett's esophagus. Gastrointest Endosc 35:442–443, 1989.

25. Silverman S, Shillitoe EJ. Etiology and predisposing factors. In Silverman S (ed): Oral Cancer, 2nd ed. Atlanta: American Cancer Society, 1985, pp. 7–36.

26. Parkin SM, Laara E, Muir CS. Estimates of the worldwide frequency of sixteen major cancers. Int J Cancer 41:184–197, 1988.

27. Baden E. Tabac et cancers de la region oropharyngee et des bronches. Donnees actuelles. Revue de Medecine de Toulouse 14:549–560, 1978.

28. Dunham LJ. A geographic study of a relationship between oral cancer and plants. Cancer Res 28:2369–2371, 1968.

29. U.S. Department of Health and Human Services: The Health Consequences of Smoking & Cancer, 1982. A report of the Surgeon General. DHS Publication No. 82-5017, 1982.

30. Ziegler RG. A review of epidemiologic evidence that carotenoids reduce the risk of cancer. J Nutr 119:116–122, 1989.

31. Burge-Bottenbley A, Shklar G. Retardation of experimental oral cancer development by retinyl acetate. Nutr Cancer 5:121–129, 1983.

32. Schwartz J, Suda D, Light G. Beta-carotene is associated with the regression of hamster buccal pouch carcinoma and induction of tumor necrosis factor in macrophages. Biochem Biophys Res Commun 136:1130–1135, 1986.

33. Shklar G, Schwartz J, Trickler D, Reid S. Regression of experimental cancer by oral administration of combined alpha-tocopherol and beta-carotene. Nutr Cancer 12:321–325, 1989.

34. Stich HF, Rosin MP, Hornby AP, Mathew B. Remission of oral leukoplakias and micronuclei in tobacco/betel quid chewers treated with beta-carotene and with beta-carotene plus vitamin A. Int J Cancer 42:195–199, 1988.

35. Karp DD, Guralnick E, Guidice LA, Meuser C, Vaughan CW, Faling LJ, Levine JD, Hong WK. Multiple primary cancers: A prevalent and increasing problem. Proceedings of the American Society of Clinical Oncology 4:13, 1985.
36. Kotwall C, Razack MS, Sako K, Rao U. Multiple primary cancers in squamous cell cancers of the head and neck. J Surg Oncol 40:97–99, 1990.
37. McGuirt WF, Mathew B, Kaufman JA. Multiple simultaneous tumors in patients with head and neck cancer. Cancer 50:1195–1199, 1982.
38. Wong F, Epstein J, Millner A. Treatment of oral leukoplakia with topical bleomycin. Cancer 64:361–365, 1989.
39. Koch HF. Biochemical treatment of precancerous oral lesions: The effectiveness of various analogues of retinoic acid. J Oral Surg 6:59–63, 1978.
40. Hong WK, Endicott J, Itri LM, Doos W, Batsakis JG, Bell R, Fofonoff S, Byers R, Atkinson EN, Vaughan C, Toth BB, Kramer A, Dimery IW, Skipper P, Strong S. 13-Cis retinoic acid in the treatment of oral leukoplakia. N Engl J Med 315:1501–1505, 1986.
41. Stich HF, Hornby AP, Mathew B, Sankaranarayanan R, Nair MK. Response of oral leukoplakias to the administration of vitamin A. Cancer Lett 40:93–101, 1988.
42. Garewal HS, Meyskens FL, Killen D, Reeves D, Kiersch TA, Elletson H, Strosberg A, King D, Steinbronn K. Response of oral leukoplakia to beta-carotene. J Clin Oncol 8:1715–1720, 1990.
43. Reid BJ, Haggitt RC, Rubin CE, Roth G, Surawicz CM, Van Belle G, Lewin K, Weinstein WM, Antonioli DA, Goldman H, MacDonald W, Owen D. Observer variation in the diagnosis of dysplasia in Barrett's esophagus. Human Pathol 19:166–178, 1988.
44. Crissman JD. The pathology of incipient neoplasia. In Henson ED, Albores-Saavedra J (eds): Upper Aerodigestive Tract. Philadelphia: WB Saunders, 1986, pp. 39–55.

Carotene and Retinol Efficacy Trial: Lung Cancer Chemoprevention Trial in Heavy Cigarette Smokers and Asbestos-exposed Workers

Gary E. Goodman, Gilbert S. Omenn, and CARET Coinvestigators and Staff

Swedish Hospital Tumor Institute
Fred Hutchinson Cancer Research Center
University of Washington
Seattle, Washington

INTRODUCTION

Lung cancer is a major cause of cancer mortality in the United States, with an estimated 143,000 deaths in 1991. In males, the rate of increase in lung cancer deaths has slowed, but the mortality rate still surpasses that of any other cancer. In females, the annual number of deaths continues to climb, and lung cancer now surpasses breast cancer as the leading cause of death (1).

The etiologic agent has been well described. Studies in the early 1950s showed a clear relationship between lung cancer mortality rates and cigarette use (2). This has focused prevention efforts on ways to discontinue or decrease smoking. However, compared with nonsmokers, even those smokers who stop smoking continue to have an increased risk of developing lung cancer (3,4).

Another characteristic of lung cancer is the tendency for diagnosis to occur late in the natural history of the disease. Most patients present with unresectable disease, and those whose disease is resectable have a high incidence of both local recurrence and disseminated disease. Once diagnosed, the therapeutic modalities of radiation therapy and combination chemotherapy have made little impact on survival.

These features make lung cancer a promising target for chemoprevention strategies. It is a common disease causing major mortality, it has a well-described causative exposure, and current therapy is poor. Clearly, any success in preventing this disease would be a major public health advantage.

CHEMOPREVENTION AGENTS

Animal studies utilizing naturally occurring and carcinogen-induced malignancies have shown that retinol and its family of naturally occurring and synthetic congeners (the retinoids) are effective in delaying or preventing the emergence of malignant tumors (5). Epidemiologic studies have suggested inverse relationships between serum concentrations of β-carotene (and

The Biology and Prevention of Aerodigestive Tract Cancers
Edited by G.R.Newell and W.K. Hong, Plenum Press, New York, 1992

137

retinol) and lung cancer incidence (6). Although extensive human trials have not been completed, a few trials studying intermediate end points and second primaries have shown promising results. In 1982, Gouveia et al. showed that etretinate decreased the metaplastic changes in the bronchial biopsy of 11 heavy smokers (7). Hong et al. studied 13-*cis*–retinoic acid in patients with early-stage squamous cell carcinoma of the head and neck and showed a decrease in the incidence of secondary primaries (8). These trials suggest that retinoids can reverse preneoplastic changes in the bronchus and decrease malignant transformation in the oral pharyngeal cavity.

INTERVENTION TRIALS AND PHASE II TRIALS

A major consideration in planning a chemoprevention trial in a population of smokers who have only an increased cancer risk is, ironically, their good health. This group does not regard themselves as ill. They may not be seeing a physician, and frequently, they may have little contact with the medical care system. Since these populations are generally asymptomatic, any agent causing significant or frequent side effects would likely not be tolerated. Continued adherence to a chemoprevention agent requires that the agent have a very low incidence of side effects. Thus, we felt that it would be unlikely that any of the synthetic retinoids would be desirable agents in this target population. On the other hand, β-carotene and retinol appear to have had an acceptable spectrum of side effects.

Based on the literature available, in 1985 we initiated a Phase II pilot trial in two high-risk populations (9), smokers and occupationally exposed asbestos workers. The smokers' pilot trial investigated β-carotene (30 mg/day) and retinol (25,000 U/day) in a 2 × 2 design; 1029 participants were randomized. In the asbestos-exposed workers' trial, the combination of β-carotene (15 mg/day) plus retinol (25,000 U/day) was compared with the placebo. In that trial, 816 participants were randomized. Besides evaluating methods of recruitment and retention rates, we focused on monitoring side effects. Thirteen symptoms and signs were monitored via a standardized questionnaire and physical examination at 2–4-month intervals. At each contact, participants were graded on a standardized grading scale for the presence and intensity of each symptom.

With follow-up through 6/30/91, these agents have been well tolerated. The only difference seen between assigned treatments has been mild yellow skin color in the groups receiving β-carotene. No significant difference was seen over time or between treatment groups for SGOT, alkaline phosphatase, cholesterol, or triglycerides.

β-CAROTENE AND RETINOL EFFICACY TRIAL (CARET)

Because recruitment goals were met, these agents appeared to be well tolerated and adherence was high (medication rate was approximately 70% at 3 years). The National Cancer Institute approved our proposal for a full-scale trial (10), evaluating the efficacy of these agents.

To maintain vigilance against potential long-term side effects, the original treatment arms of the pilot trials were revised so that participants receiving placebos remained on placebos and those receiving any active agent were combined into one treatment group consisting of β-carotene (30 mg/day) and retinyl palmitate (25,000 U/day) (Figure). The smokers and the asbestos-exposed pilot populations were combined to make up the vanguard population. Follow-up on the vanguard population is at 3-month intervals, with close monitoring of serum parameters and 13 subjective and objective symptoms potentially related to these compounds. This group is followed, in parallel, with a larger, newly recruited population that will eventually make up 90% of the CARET population. Because side effects to these agents may

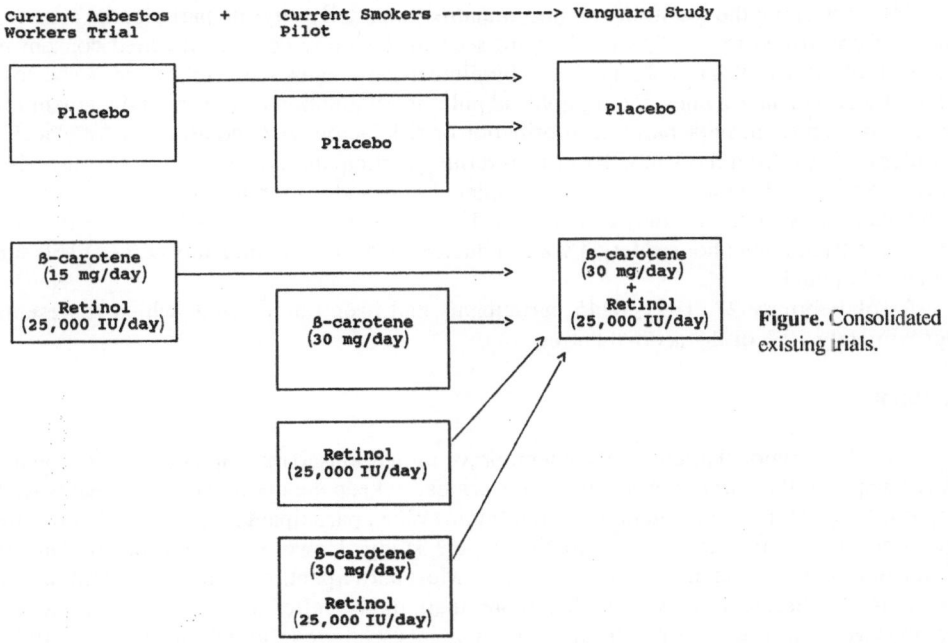

```
Current Asbestos     +     Current Smokers -----------> Vanguard Study
Workers Trial              Pilot
```

Figure. Consolidated existing trials.

be related to cumulative dosage, it is expected that any side effect related to these agents will occur in the vanguard population initially. The close monitoring of the vanguard group allows a less-intensive monitoring and more cost-effective follow-up of the larger efficacy population.

Additional recruitment to CARET was initiated in June 1989. CARET is a multicenter collaboration with a recruitment goal of 4277 asbestos workers and 13,629 smokers (10). All participants will be randomized to β-carotene (30 mg/day) plus retinyl palmitate (25,000 U/day), in one capsule or to placebo. Participants will be monitored for medication rate, side effects, end points of lung cancer, other cancers, and cause of death.

The smoking population is being recruited via the mailing of recruitment materials to age-selected subscribers of major health insurance carriers. Smokers are being recruited by principal investigators from Seattle, Washington (Gary E. Goodman, P.I.); Portland, Oregon (Barbara Valanis, P.I.); and Irvine, California (Frank Meyskens, P.I.). Asbestos-exposed workers are recruited via workmen's compensation insurance systems, pulmonary and occupational medicine clinics, union rolls, and other sources. This population is being recruited from San Francisco, California (Jim Balmer, P.I.); New London, Connecticut (Mark Cullen, P.I.); and Baltimore, Maryland (James Keogh, P.I.), as well as Portland and Seattle.

Eligibility criteria for the smoker population are age (50–69 years), a smoking history (>20 pack-years), and status as current smokers or ex-smokers (quit <6 years ago). Eligibility criteria for asbestos-exposed workers include the following: men aged 45–69 years, current smokers or ex-smokers (quit <15 years ago), and extensive occupational exposure to asbestos, which includes 15 years or more since the first exposure and an abnormal chest X ray compatible with asbestos exposure by International Labour Organisation criteria or 5 years or more in a defined high-risk trade, or both.

Participants are excluded from the study when there is a history of cancer within the previous 5 years, when there are elevated levels of SGOT or alkaline phosphatase (>2.5 or 1.5 times the 95th percentile of normal, respectively), or when they are taking vitamin A (<5500 IU/day) or any β-carotene supplements.

After returning the recruitment questionnaire, potentially eligible participants are contacted. If confirmed to be eligible, they are seen in the study center, informed consent is obtained, blood samples are obtained, and baseline questionnaires are completed. Asbestos-exposed workers have a chest radiograph and pulmonary function tests as an inducement for participation and to provide baseline information on risk factors. A 3-month supply of placebo capsules is given. After the 3-month run-in, returning participants are randomized to the active study agents. A telephone interview is completed at 3 and 9 months from randomization. Participants are seen in the study center 6 and 12 months from randomization. After the first year of the trial, a telephone interview is conducted twice a year and study center visits are conducted annually.

As of February 28, 1991, 6245 participants had been randomized, which represents approximately 70% of the accrual target.

Retention

One of the major challenges of a chemoprevention trial is to maintain participants on the study agents for the duration of the trial. It is critical to keep the number of participants who drop out (stop taking study agents) to a minimum. When participants join CARET, they are interested and excited to be participating in the study. However, over time, it appears participants lose this initial level of excitement. Most participants cite minor problems as the reason for withdrawal; however, this more than likely reflects study fatigue. Many chemoprevention trials will be recruiting participants who are relatively healthy. It will be critical to cultivate the interest and enthusiasm of the participants to maintain long-term retention.

REFERENCES

1. Boring C, Squires T, Tong T. Cancer statistics. CA 41:19–36, 1991.
2. Hammond EC, Horn D. Smoking and death rates: Report on 44 months of follow-up of 187,783 men. II. Death rates by cancer. JAMA 166:1294–1308, 1958.
3. Lubin JH, Blot WJ, Berrino F, Flamant R, Gillis CR, Kunze M, Schmahl D, Visco G. Modifying risk of developing lung cancer by changing habits of cigarette smoking. Br Med J 288:1953–1956, 1984.
4. Doll R, Peto J. Mortality in relation to smoking: 20 Years' observation on male British doctors. Br Med J 2:1525–1536, 1976.
5. Byers T: Diet and cancer: Any progress in the "interim"? Presented at the Second National Conference on Cancer Prevention and Detection. Seattle, Washington, 1987.
6. Bertram J, Kolonel L, Meyskens F. Rationale and strategies for chemoprevention of cancer in humans. Cancer Res 47:3012–3031, 1987.
7. Gouveia J, Mathe G, Hercend T, Gros F, Lemaigre G, Santelli G, Homasson JP, Gaillard JP, Angebault M, Bonnoit JP, Lededente A, Marsac J, Parrot R, Pretet S. Degree of bronchial metaplasia in heavy smokers and its regression after treatment with a retinoid. Lancet 1:710–712, 1982.
8. Hong WK, Lippman SM, Itri LM, Karp DD, Lee JS, Byers RM, Schantz SP, Kramer AM, Lotan R, Peters LJ, Dimery IW, Brown BW, Goepfert H. Prevention of second primary tumors with isotretinoin in squamous cell carcinoma of the head and neck. N Engl J Med 20:795–800, 1990.
9. Omenn GS. A double-blind randomized trial with beta-carotene and retinol in persons at high risk of lung cancer due to occupational asbestos exposure and/or cigarette smoking. Public Health Rev 16:99–125, 1988.
10. Grizzle J, Omenn G, Goodman G, Thornquist M, Barnhart S, Balmes J, Cherniak M, Cone J, Cullen M, Glass A, Keogh J, Valanis B. Design of the beta-carotene and retinol efficacy trial (CARET) for chemoprevention of cancer in populations at high risk: Heavy smokers and asbestos-exposed workers. Presented at the First International Conference on Chemoprevention of Cancer. Vienna, Austria, August 1990.

An Intervention Trial in High-Risk Asbestos-exposed Persons

Jerry W. McLarty

Department of Epidemiology/Biomathematics
The University of Texas Health Science Center at Tyler
Tyler, Texas

INTRODUCTION

Lung cancer, the treatment of which is essentially no more effective today than it was 20 years ago, remains the major cause of cancer mortality in the United States, killing more than 140,000 persons annually. Persons who are occupationally exposed to asbestos are at extremely high risk for lung cancer, from 10 to 50 or more times higher than normal—depending upon their smoking history. In the following discussion, we present the study design for an ongoing intervention trial among 750 asbestos workers in Tyler, Texas. β-Carotene and retinol are being used as the chemopreventive agents and an intermediate end point, sputum atypia, as the measure of response. Some results of baseline data analysis (before initiation of treatment) will be presented below. Findings of toxicity, recruitment, and compliance will also be discussed.

ASBESTOS AND LUNG CANCER

Asbestos is a relatively inert mineral fiber whose airborne particles can be deposited in the respiratory tract by a variety of mechanisms and can remain there for many years. Persons exposed to occupational levels of asbestos are at high risk for at least four distinct diseases: fibrotic lung disease (asbestosis), bronchogenic cancer, nonmalignant pleural disease, and mesothelioma. It appears that the highly durable asbestos fiber may act as both a tumor initiator and promoter (1,2). Furthermore, lung cancer risk in asbestos workers is significantly increased by cigarette smoking. Unfortunately, the majority of asbestos workers are smokers or have been for most of their lives. In an early study of the participants in the clinical trial described below, 85% had a history of smoking (3). The asbestos exposure of the Tyler workers was very heavy, with measured dust levels hundreds of times higher than the standards later enforced by government regulating agencies.

β-CAROTENE AND RETINOL

For cancer chemoprevention, trials must use agents that have at least a demonstrated potential for efficacy and levels of toxicity that can be managed in a clinical trial setting for

The Biology and Prevention of Aerodigestive Tract Cancers
Edited by G.R.Newell and W.K. Hong, Plenum Press, New York, 1992

141

reasonable periods of time. When most of the ongoing clinical chemoprevention trials were initiated, the evidence for efficacy was predominantly from a large number of case-control and prospective epidemiologic studies. The epidemiologic studies, especially for lung cancer, were strikingly consistent from study to study in many different locations around the world (4–7). Most of these studies found that diets high in fruits or vegetables, or both, were associated with a lower cancer risk. Serum studies confirmed that β-carotene and retinol were also negatively associated with cancer risk, suggesting that they might be the active anticancer (or protective) agents in the fruit and vegetable diets; laboratory and animal experiments have added support to this hypothesis.

There is abundant evidence for the antitumor properties of retinoids (vitamin A and its synthetic derivatives) (8). Retinoids have been shown to suppress malignant transformations and tumor promotion, to delay or prevent the onset of cancer in experimental animals, and even to reverse the process of carcinogenesis (9). Vitamin A has been used in therapeutic clinical trials of people with cancer in both its natural (10,11) and synthetic forms (12). However, the prophylactic or chemopreventive use of retinoids in humans may be limited by the excessive toxicity owing to hypervitaminosis (13). Retinol has been used safely at very high doses administered over short periods of time (14); but the safety of long-term low doses, as required for an intervention trial, remains to be determined.

β-Carotene is a vegetable precursor of vitamin A (retinol) that is converted in the intestine to the aldehyde form of vitamin A. The metabolism of β-carotene to retinol is regulated such that hypervitaminosis A does not occur, even when excessively high levels of β-carotene are present (15). Serum levels of β-carotene increase proportionately with dietary intake, but retinol levels do not. Moreover, animal toxicity studies and long-term human studies show no significant toxicity to high levels of β-carotene (16–18). A number of case-control studies of β-carotene serum levels or dietary intake (in which cancer cases were compared with similar controls) provide direct support for a significant protective effect of β-carotene against a variety of cancers (19–21). A recent review of 22 case-control studies (5) showed that 18 of the 22 studies found a β-carotene–rich diet to be associated with a decreased risk for epithelial cell cancer at eight different sites. Especially relevant to this proposal of a protective effect was the observation that β-carotene was found to be the most promising of four micronutrients studied in a recent case-control study (22). Prospective dietary and serum studies have shown similar correlations between low β-carotene intake and subsequent high risk of cancer (23–25).

The relevance of β-carotene to preneoplastic conditions (as in the current study of sputum atypias), and not just carcinoma, was shown in a case-control dietary study of cervical dysplasia (26) in which a significant β-carotene protective effect was found. Also relevant to the present Tyler study, Wahi et al. (20) found low serum levels of β-carotene in patients with leukoplakia and oral cancer. Further, there was a consistent trend toward lower carotene levels in the progressively higher levels of atypia (e.g., grades II–IV). A similar trend of decreasing serum carotene levels at increasing levels of dysplasia and cancer has been demonstrated with cervical dysplasia (22). Also recently, Stich et al. (27) have shown that both β-carotene and retinol can reduce the proportion of micronucleated mucosal cells, cells thought to be related to an increased risk for cancer and which may represent a preneoplastic condition. We have shown that the presence of micronuclei in sputum is significantly associated with sputum atypia (28).

The possible mechanisms for the anticancer effects of β-carotene may include direct antioxidant/radical scavenging properties (29,30), enhancement of the host immune response (31,32), decrease in DNA damage by carcinogens (33), and inducement of morphologic differentiation of cells by alteration of the adenylate cyclase system (34).

Reasons for using both β-carotene and retinol include the following: (a) Epidemiologic evidence strongly suggests an epithelial anticancer effect for β-carotene, as well as for retinoids. (b) β-carotene is converted to retinol in the intestine, to a degree, and therefore can support retinoid effects. If both agents are given simultaneously, it is possible that less of the β-carotene will be converted and result in higher serum carotene levels. (c) The two agents have some mechanisms of action that may be independent, so giving both simultaneously may have an enhanced chemopreventive effect.

SPUTUM CYTOLOGY

One unique feature of the present study is the use of a putative intermediate cancer end point, atypical sputum cytopathology, as the measure of response to the intervention drugs. Sputum atypia is believed to reflect bronchial dysplasia (a preneoplastic lesion or at least an intermediate marker of lung cancer risk). As discussed below, sputum atypia is highly prevalent in asbestos workers, is shown to be inversely related to serum β-carotene, and is a significant risk factor for lung cancer in asbestos workers.

Atypical and malignant cells are found concurrently in both histologic and sputum specimens from lung cancer patients (35). Studies of uranium miners and experimental animals have indicated that sputum squamous metaplasia is often a precursor of neoplasia, particularly in patients with marked atypia (36). In our own experience with the Tyler asbestos workers, we found that moderate atypia or greater in a single sputum specimen was a significant risk factor for the subsequent development of lung cancer (37). Regression analysis has shown that in asbestos workers—at least those exposed to amosite asbestos—lung cancer and sputum atypia have the same risk factors (i.e., age, asbestos exposure, and smoking) in a qualitatively similar fashion (38). The increasing cellular alterations at higher levels of atypia are thought to be reversible (36).

Carotene levels have been found to correlate (inversely) with dysplasia at other epidermoid sites. Cervical dysplasia was related to low dietary and serum β-carotene, as described previously (22,26); oral leukoplakias were found to be significantly correlated with low serum β-carotene (20). We found that low serum levels of β-carotene were significantly related to the degree of sputum atypia in asbestos workers (39).

Cervical dysplasia, bronchial metaplasia, and oral leukoplakia have been successfully treated (i.e., prevented) in humans, and bronchial dysplasia has been prevented in animal models with β-carotene and retinol. It is believed that sputum atypia is analogous to these dysplastic epithelial lesions and that the drugs have the potential to lower the incidence and prevalence of sputum atypia in asbestos workers.

Perhaps the most important reason for using sputum atypia as the end point in an intervention trial is that it is the only noninvasive means of monitoring the contents of the lungs. As a highly prevalent finding in asbestos workers, it can be monitored repeatedly, with a much smaller sample size than for lung cancer incidence and mortality, the traditional lung cancer end points.

PROTOCOL DESCRIPTION

Study Design

The ongoing Tyler study is a randomized, double-blind, placebo-controlled clinical trial of two agents, β-carotene and retinol. Persons who are occupationally exposed to asbestos are being used as subjects, and sputum atypia is the primary study end point. The overall schema is to examine patients initially, put those who qualify on the placebo for a 6-week run-in period, and then randomize those who successfully complete the run-in period to one of two arms: β-carotene (50 mg/day) and retinol (25,000 IU on alternate days) or placebo. The duration of treatment was initially planned to be 3 years, but a renewal of the study allowed recruitment of additional subjects and an extension of time for the original recruits. The minimum time on drug for any participant will be 3 years; the maximum, 6 years.

Study Population

The particular cohort of Tyler asbestos workers was chosen for the described clinical trial for several reasons: they were available to the investigators because of a long-term relationship with the institution (3); they were documented to have exceptionally high levels of asbestos exposure; and they were shown to have a high prevalence of sputum atypia, the specific end point for the study (40). However, to recruit a sufficient number of participants for the clinical trial, the Tyler group was augmented with asbestos workers in other industries in Texas.

Persons with any of the following conditions were excluded from participation: preexisting liver or kidney disease, abnormal liver function tests (>2.5 times normal values), active lung cancer or radiographic findings suggestive of cancer, childbearing potential.

Randomization

Before randomization, patients were stratified by four known risk factors for lung cancer and sputum atypia: place of employment, age, smoking, and time since first asbestos exposure. The goal of stratification was to achieve an initial balance of sputum atypia in the two drug groups.

Drug Administration

Drugs are packaged in monthly calendar packs with the appropriate daily dose under individual blisters in the calendar packs: β-carotene (50 mg/day of BASF β-carotene capsules) and retinol (25,000 IU, taken on alternate days). The duration of treatment, depending upon when the patients entered the study, will be from 3 to 6 years. If the patients are unable to tolerate the assigned dose, the regimen will be modified by the clinical administrator on an individual basis, as described later.

Assessment of Smoking and Nutritional Status

Smoking and tobacco-use information are obtained from a standardized questionnaire (41), which was modified to include questions concerning the use of snuff and chewing tobacco. More important, two serum measurements of smoking (cotinine and thiocyanate) are obtained at each visit.

A nutrient estimation instrument developed by Dr. Gladys Block (42) from the Division of Cancer Prevention and Control, National Cancer Institute (Bethesda, MD), has been used. This questionnaire can be completed quickly by an interview at examination time.

Sample-Size Estimation

Sample-size estimates were computed to achieve a one-third reduction in the percentage of atypical-sputum specimens in the active-drug group as compared with the placebo group. Type I and II error probabilities of 0.05 and 0.2, respectively, were used. Assuming a loss of 30% due to causes such as death, dropout, and toxicity, at least 600 randomized patients would be required.

Patient Management

Examinations and Assays. (a) A routine physical examination is performed every 6 months, including chest radiographs (at 2-year intervals, or as otherwise indicated), listening for chest sounds, checking for clubbing, edema, liver, and kidney pathology. The purposes of the examination are to screen for cancer, to document asbestos-related disease, to serve as an initial recruitment incentive, and to monitor protocol-related toxicity.

(b) Routine liver function tests, including serum bilirubin, SGOT, and alkaline phosphatase (first visit, semiannually thereafter) are done as part of the routine patient evaluation and to monitor for hepatic toxicity.

(c) Serum lipids are tested at first visit, at 6 weeks, and semiannually thereafter since serum cholesterol and triglycerides have been shown to be correlated with serum retinol levels (43) and carotene levels (44). Potential changes owing to β-carotene administration are also monitored.

(d) β-Carotene and retinol assays are performed at first visit, 6 weeks after start of therapy, and semiannually thereafter to monitor patient compliance and to measure the effects of long-term β-carotene administration on serum levels.

(e) All sputum specimens are processed for cytologic examination by the Saccomanno homogenization technique and stained by the Papanicolaou method (36). Two distinct collection methods are used: (i) induction of sputum discharge by hypertonic saline aerosol administered with an ultrasonic nebulizer (first visit, at 6 weeks, and semiannually thereafter), and (ii) spontaneous discharge, pooled from early-morning cough on 3 successive days (collected immediately after initial and semiannual visits and every 3 months thereafter). Spontaneous specimens are sent in by prepaid mail.

Patients with Positive Findings. Patients with sputum positive for cancer cells have the sputum test repeated immediately. After verification, patients are removed from β-carotene or placebo, and hospitalization for tumor localization and treatment is offered. Serum is collected for the clinical trial at this time. As with all patients withdrawn from the study, cancer patients' data are returned for inclusion in the final analysis. Patients found to have severe atypia are followed more frequently and, at the clinical administrator's discretion, are offered bronchoscopy or other more intensive clinical evaluations. These patients are not routinely removed from the protocol.

Toxicity Management. A five-level scale (grades 0–4) has been devised for signs and symptoms related to possible retinol toxicity. Four basic categories are evaluated: dermatologic, metabolic, behavioral, and blood chemistries. Within each category, there are a number of related toxicity measures (e.g., erythema) that are graded for each patient by the nurse clinicians. A score of 3 or greater on any toxicity measure will result in a patient being entered into the toxicity-management/dose-modification cascade. The plan is to first remove retinol (or retinol placebo) from the treatment for patients with suspected toxicity. If this is not sufficient to lower toxic levels, β-carotene (or β-carotene placebo) is then removed. Various strategies are used to rule out problems not related to the protocol and to put patients back on the protocol if at all possible.

RESULTS

Since the study has 2 more years remaining, no end point results are yet reportable. However, the early recruiting, baseline data analysis, and toxicity reporting are discussed below.

Patient Recruitment

The recruitment process involved an initial visit, a 6-week placebo run-in period, and randomization of eligible patients. More than 1100 persons were screened to identify eligible participants; 758 successfully completed the run-in period and were randomized onto the drug protocol. Most dropouts left the study during the first 6-month interval between examinations, and the study population remained remarkably stable after that. This suggests that a run-in period longer than 6 weeks may have resulted in fewer dropouts.

Baseline Data Analysis

The average age at randomization was 52 years. Ninety-five percent of the randomized applicants were men. Seventy-seven percent were white, 22% black, and the remainder Hispanic or Asian, a distribution that closely resembled the general population in our catchment area. Most of the participants were current or ex-smokers: 38% were current smokers; 42.5% were ex-smokers; and 19.5% had never smoked.

The figure shows the distribution of sputum cytopathology diagnoses before randomization with the expected unusually high prevalence of sputum atypia.

The prerandomization mean serum β-carotene level was 189 ng/ml (standard deviation ± 185), lower than reported in most other series of patients (45) using similar assay methods. The low serum levels emphasize the high risk of this particular cohort: the workers are at high risk for lung cancer because of their asbestos and cigarette-smoking exposures, and perhaps additionally because of their low-serum β-carotene levels. Serum retinol levels were essentially normal at baseline, 590 ng/ml. The serum β-carotene levels rose to roughly 10 times baseline levels for those taking the active drugs (mean of 1816 ng/ml after 12 months on drugs).

Compliance

Compliance is being monitored by three mechanisms: self-reports, capsule counts, and β-carotene serum levels. According to the self-reports, 95% of participants said they took the drugs most of the time. This agrees with a 93% estimated compliance rate from the capsule counts. There is a wide range of serum levels, with considerable overlap in the distributions of the two drug groups. Taking the upper seventy-fifth percentile of the placebo group as a reference point, it was found that 14.4% of the active drug group has serum levels as low or lower. The results of the compliance measure analysis suggest that between 86 and 93% of the patients are reasonably compliant with the protocol.

Figure. Prevalence of pretreatment sputum atypia (highest of first two visits). The most atypical speci-men of four preran-domization speci-mens was used for each participant. The "active"-drug group is receiving β-caro-tene and retinol.

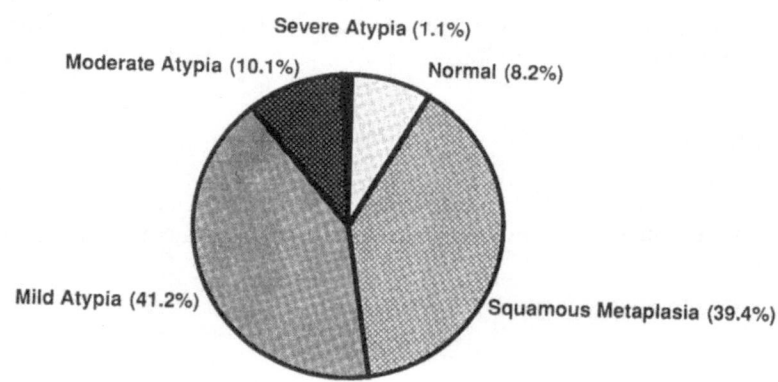

Table. Serum Vitamin E Comparisons Between Active-Drug and Placebo Groups

Months Since Randomization	Serum Vitamin E (μg/ml)	
	Active-Drug Group	Placebo Group
0	13.8	12.6
12	14.3	11.3
48	14.3	13.0

Toxicity

Toxicity monitoring consists of clinic visits with physical examinations, serum lipid analysis, liver and kidney function tests, and a questionnaire specifically designed to record possible retinol side effects. There have been reports of symptoms that could be related to toxicity such as headache, skin dryness, and chapped lips. However, except for skin yellowing, there is no significant difference in the frequency of symptoms between active-drug and placebo groups. With one exception, no differences have been observed in any of the laboratory measures. Early in the study, a statistically significant increase in mean serum triglycerides was observed in the active-drug group: 193 mg/dl in the active-drug group versus 167 mg/dl in the placebo group. However, no patient reached clinically alarming levels, and recent indications are that the active-drug group levels are now reverting to original levels. As shown in the table, there was no difference in the serum vitamin E levels between groups after many months on β-carotene. This finding contradicts a preliminary report of decreases in serum vitamin E after 12 months of β-carotene therapy in another chemoprevention trial (46). However, the studies are not strictly comparable since the Tyler protocol includes both retinol and β-carotene.

SUMMARY AND DISCUSSION

In this chapter, a rationale has been presented for the use of β-carotene and retinol in an intervention trial with high-risk asbestos workers. The use of sputum atypia as an intermediate marker or preneoplastic lesion has been proposed. The currently ongoing study described above appears to have satisfactorily met its recruitment goals and protocol adherence requirements. No significant toxicity has been demonstrated with the prescribed doses of β-carotene and retinol, even after several years of use. It is hoped that the drugs, dosage, duration of treatment, and study design and execution will be sufficient for a definitive conclusion at the end of the trial.

REFERENCES

1. Rom WN, Travis WD, Brody AR. Cellular and molecular basis of the asbestos-related diseases. Am Rev Respir Dis 143:408–422, 1991.
2. Jaurand MC. Particulate–state carcinogenesis: A survey of recent studies on the mechanisms of action of fibres. IARC Sci Publ 90:54–73, 1989.
3. Hurst GA, Spivey CG, Matlage WT, Miller JM, Faulk G, Hieger LR, McLarty JW, Greenberg SD. The Tyler Asbestos Workers Program: I. A medical surveillance model and method. Arch Environ Health 34:432–439, 1979.
4. Mayne ST. Beta-carotene and cancer prevention: What is the evidence? Conn Med 54:547–551, 1990.
5. Hennekens CH. Micronutrients and cancer prevention (editorial). N Engl J Med 315:1288–1289, 1986.
6. Hennekens CH. Vitamin A analogues in cancer chemoprevention. Important Adv Oncol 1986:23–35, 1986.

7. Fontham ETH. Protective dietary factors and lung cancer. Int J Epidemiol 19:S32–S42, 1990.
8. Sporn MB, Newton DL. Chemoprevention of cancer with retinoids. Federal Proceedings 38:2528–2534, 1979.
9. Bolag W, Matter A. From vitamin A to retinoids in experimental and clinical oncology: Achievements, failures and outlook. Ann N Y Acad Sci 359:9–21, 1981.
10. Meyskens FL, Moon TE, Alberts DS, Bowden GT, Earnest DL. Vitamin A Program Project, ICRDB, Protocol No. PO1 CA 27502 (NCI Grant).
11. Alth G. Aspects of the immunologic treatment of lung cancer. Cancer Chemotherapy Reports 4:271–274, 1973.
12. Peck GL, Olsen TG, Butkus D. Treatment of basal cell carcinomas with 13-*cis*–retinoic acid (abstract). Proceedings of the American Association for Cancer Research 20:56, 1979.
13. Muenter MD, Perry MO, Ludwig J. Chronic vitamin A intoxication in adults. Am J Med 50:129–136, 1971.
14. Bauernfeind JC. The Safe Use of Vitamin A: A Report of the International Vitamin A Consultative Group. Washington, DC: The Nutrition Foundation, 1980.
15. Bagdon RE, Zbinden G, Studer A. Chronic toxicity studies of beta-carotene. Toxicol Appl Pharmacol 2:225–236, 1960.
16. Mathews-Roth M-M. Lack of genotoxicity with beta-carotene. Toxicol Lett 41:185–191, 1988.
17. Mathus VEM, Tytgat GN. Biological fate of the vitamin A transporting protein complex and beta-carotene after excessive dietary intake: Report of a case. Digestion 27:116–122, 1983.
18. Bendich A. The safety of beta-carotene. Nutr Cancer 11:207–214, 1988.
19. Atukorala S, Basu TK, Dickerson JWT. Vitamin A, zinc and lung cancer. Br J Cancer 40:927–931, 1979.
20. Wahi PN, Bodkhe RR, Arora S, Srivastava MC. Serum vitamin A studies in leukoplakia and carcinoma of the oral cavity. Indian J Pathol Bacteriol 5:10–16, 1962.
21. Mettlin C, Graham S, Swanson M. Vitamin A and lung cancer. J Natl Cancer Inst 62:1435–1438, 1979.
22. Menkes MS, Comstock GW, Vuilleumier JP, Helsing KJ, Rider AA, Brookmeyer R. Serum beta-carotene, vitamins A and E, selenium, and the risk of lung cancer. N Engl J Med 315:1250–1254, 1986.
23. Shekelle RB, Lepper M, Liu S, Maliza C, Raynor WJJ, Rossof AH, Paul O, Shryock AM, Stamler J. Dietary vitamin A and risk of cancer in the Western Electric study. Lancet 2:1186–1190, 1981.
24. Kark JD, Smith AH, Switzer BR, Hames CG. Serum vitamin A (retinol) and cancer incidence in Evans County, Georgia. J Natl Cancer Inst 66:7–16, 1981.
25. Wald NJ, Thompson SG, Densem JW, Boreham J, Bailey A. Serum beta-carotene and subsequent risk of cancer: Results from the BUPA Study. Br J Cancer 57:428–433, 1988.
26. Romney SL, Palan PR, Duttagupta C, Wassertheil-Smoller S, Wiley G, Slagle NS, Lucido D. Retinoids and the prevention of cervical dysplasias. Am J Obstet Gynecol 141:890–894, 1981.
27. Stich HF, Rosin MP, Hornby AP, Mathew B, Sankaranarayanan R, Nair MK. Remission of oral leukoplakias and micronuclei in tobacco/betel quid chewers treated with beta-carotene and with beta-carotene plus vitamin A. Int J Cancer 42:195–199, 1988.
28. Yanagihara R, Holiday D, Riley L, O'Donnell L, Mabry L, Fagan M, McLarty J. Micronucleated sputum bronchial cells: Potential intermediate end point for lung cancer (abstract). Proceedings of the American Society of Clinical Oncology 8:58, 1989.
29. Santamaria L, Bianchi A, Arnaboldi A, Ravetto C, Bianchi L, Pizzala R, Andreoni L, Santagati G, Bermond P. Chemoprevention of indirect and direct chemical carcinogenesis by carotenoids as oxygen radical quenchers. Ann N Y Acad Sci 534:584–596, 1988.
30. Mathews M, Roth M. Photoprotection by carotenoids. Federal Proceedings 46:1890–1893, 1987.
31. Abril ER, Rybski JA, Scuderi P, Watson RR. Beta-carotene stimulates human leukocytes to secrete a novel cytokine. J Leukoc Biol 45:255–261, 1989.
32. Bendich A. Antioxidant micronutrients and immune responses. Ann N Y Acad Sci 587:168–180, 1990.
33. Weitberg AB, Weitzman SA, Clark EP, Stossel TP. Effects of antioxidants on oxidant-induced sister chromatid exchange formation. J Clin Invest 75:1835–1841, 1985.
34. Hazuka MB, Edwards PJ, Newman F, Kinzie JJ, Prasad KN. Beta-carotene induces morphological differentiation and decreases adenylate cyclase activity in melanoma cells in culture. J Am Coll Nutr 9:143–149, 1990.
35. Melamed MR, Zaman MB, Flehinger BJ, Martini N. Radiologically occult in situ and incipient invasive epidermoid lung cancer. Am J Surg Pathol 1:5–16, 1977.
36. Saccomanno G, Archer VE, Auerback O, Saunders RP, Brennan LM. Development of carcinoma of the lung as reflected in exfoliated cells. Cancer 33:256–270, 1974.
37. Yanagihara RH, McLarty J, Hieger LR, Hurst G, Greenberg SD, Mabry L, Farley M. The predictive value of sputum bronchial atypia in subjects at risk for lung cancer (abstract). Proceedings of the American Society of Clinical Oncology 6:166, 1987.
38. Whittemore AS, McLarty JW, Fortson N, Anderson K. Regression analysis of cytopathological data. Biometrics 38:899–905, 1982.
39. McLarty JW, Yanagihara RH, Riley L. Characteristics of subjects with high and low serum beta-carotene: Implications for lung cancer risk (abstract). Proceedings of the American Society of Clinical Oncology 6:A897, 1987.

40. McLarty JW, Yanagihara RH, James HL, Riley L, Kummet TD, Smith K. Baseline data analysis of serum beta-carotene in a randomized clinical trial: The Tyler Cancer Prevention Program (abstract). Chest 91:301, 1987.
41. Ferris BG. Epidemiology Standardization Project, Part II. Am Rev Respir Dis 118:6, 1978.
42. Block G, Coyle L, Harvin A, Kessler L. A dietary and risk factor questionnaire and analysis system for personal computers. Am J Epidemiol 129:445–449, 1989.
43. Basu TK, Raven RW, Dickerson JWT, Williams DC. Vitamin A nutrition and its relationship with plasma cholesterol level in the patients with cancer. Int J Vitam Nutr Res 44:14–18, 1974.
44. Willet WC, Polk BF, Underwood BA, Meir MJ, Pressel S, Bosner B, Taylor O, Schneider EK, Hames C. Relation of serum vitamins A and E and carotenoids to the risk of cancer. N Engl J Med 310:430–434, 1984.
45. Nierenberg DW, Stukel TA, Baron JA, Dain BJ, Greenberg ER. Determinants of plasma levels of beta-carotene and retinol: Skin Cancer Prevention Study Group. Am J Epidemiol 130:511–521, 1989.
46. Xu MJ, Peng YM, Liu Y, Alberts DS, Plezia PM, Sayers SW. Effect of chronic administration of beta-carotene on plasma alpha-tocopherol concentrations in normal subjects (abstract). Proceedings of the American Association for Cancer Research 31:126, 1990.

Chemoprevention of Aerodigestive Epithelial Cancers

Scott M. Lippman and Waun Ki Hong

Section of Head, Neck and Thoracic Medical Oncology
Department of Medical Oncology
The University of Texas M. D. Anderson Cancer Center
Houston, Texas

INTRODUCTION

Head and neck cancer, together with cancers of the esophagus and lung, will cause one third of all 1990 cancer deaths in the United States, or 160,000 deaths (1). The magnitude of this problem directly relates to the magnitude of tobacco use, since tobacco is the single causative agent linking these three aerodigestive tract cancers. Despite intensified attention to smoking cessation programs, tobacco continues to be a major public health problem throughout the world. Worldwide tobacco use statistics include 1 billion smokers and 600 million chewers; U.S. figures are 50 million smokers and 12 billion chewers.

During the past 20–30 years, only marginal improvement has occurred in the overall survival of patients with squamous cell carcinoma (SCC) of the head and neck (1). This improvement has been disappointing even though the primary tumors can now be controlled by the standard therapy of either surgery and/or radiotherapy or therapy incorporating neo-adjuvant chemotherapy (2). Even after successful primary therapy of early-stage or locally advanced SCC, 30–50% of patients develop local or regional recurrences, 20–30% develop distant metastases, and 10–40% develop second primary tumors (3). Within this disease, second primaries occur at a constant rate per year and are the major cause of treatment failure in patients with early-stage disease. Clearly, new strategies are needed to control this neoplastic process (4).

With their classic 1953 report on oral cancer, Slaughter et al. (5) opened the door for modern research into the chemoprevention of head and neck cancer. They realized that the entire epithelial surface exposed to repeated carcinogenic insults (e.g., from tobacco use) was at risk and suggested that this exposure increased the likelihood that multiple, independent pre-malignant and malignant foci would develop in the exposed epithelium. This concept of "field cancerization" postulates a basic pathogenic mechanism that links the primary carcinogenic process to the development of second primaries in the head and neck, esophagus, and lung (4).

This review summarizes the current status of investigation in the area of chemoprevention in the upper aerodigestive tract. We shall focus on retinoids, a class of pharmacologic agents considered to be prototypical differentiation agents, since the vast majority of preclinical and clinical chemoprevention studies involve this group of agents. Furthermore, since work in head and neck chemoprevention has focused on the oral cavity, we shall concentrate on this site.

The Biology and Prevention of Aerodigestive Tract Cancers
Edited by G.R.Newell and W.K. Hong, Plenum Press, New York, 1992

EPIDEMIOLOGY AND CARCINOGENESIS

Approximately 90% of head and neck cancers are squamous cell in origin and occur in individuals exposed to known upper aerodigestive tract carcinogens. The first case-control study linking oral SCC to tobacco and alcohol consumption appeared over 30 years ago. Tobacco, either smoked or chewed, is the major risk factor for the development of SCC of the oral cavity. A relatively weak carcinogen, tobacco initiates carcinogenesis in the head and neck in a linear dose-response fashion, the effect increasing with the amount and duration of use.

The striking regional and cultural variations in oral cancer sites and incidence are related in part to differing tobacco and alcohol use patterns. In the United States, 2% of cancers are oral cancers: 21,200 new cases and 4550 deaths were projected for 1990 (1,6). In other parts of the world, oral cancer is a far greater problem. In parts of India, SCC of the hard palate is endemic because of reverse chutta (homemade cigars) smoking. In Bombay, where tobacco with pan (betel leaf, lime, catechu, and areca nut combined) is commonly used, buccal SCC accounts for 50% of all cancers (7). Cigarettes also confer a definite risk for oral SCC although to a lesser degree than smokeless tobacco. In the United States, for example, the majority of patients with oral SCC are smokers.

Ethanol in any form (beer, wine, hard liquor) is a promoter of oral carcinogenesis. It has been difficult to establish an independent effect of alcohol in oral SCC risk since most heavy drinkers smoke and the data regarding which type of alcoholic drink confers the highest risk are conflicting. The major clinical significance of alcohol consumption is that it potentiates the oral carcinogenic effect of tobacco at every level of tobacco use, although the synergistic effect is most striking at the highest levels of exposure to both (7). The effect of alcohol, therefore, is an important consideration in the etiology and prevention of oral cancer.

Tobacco and alcohol use patterns do not account for all head and neck cancers—the incidences of smoking and drinking are far greater than that of head and neck SCC. Conversely, many SCC patients have no direct exposure to either—suggesting the role of other independent risk factors. For example, recent work has implicated viral agents (herpes simplex I virus and human papillomaviruses) and genetic susceptibility in the pathogenesis of head and neck cancer (8,9). However, despite a seemingly logical link, there does not appear to be a strong association between exposure to ionizing radiation and the development of SCC of the head and neck.

Considerable epidemiologic evidence suggests that vitamin A and β-carotene are protective against epithelial neoplasia and that a deficiency of either is a risk factor for squamous upper aerodigestive tract and lung cancers (10–12). Several groups have specifically investigated the association of dietary vitamin A, β-carotene, or both, with risk for oral cancer. Winn et al., among others, have found the risk of oral SCC in women to be inversely related to the consumption of fresh fruits and vegetables (13). Serum retinol (vitamin A) and β-carotene levels are often low in patients with head and neck SCC (14). It is unclear, however, whether these low levels are important in the pathogenesis of oral SCC or whether they develop as a result of the disease process.

No definite conclusions can be drawn from these studies, since a patient's recall of dietary history is limited. Diets are complex and difficult to assess and validate; in particular, inaccuracies often result in translating dietary information from foods to nutrients. Therefore, even in suggestive epidemiologic studies such as these, it is impossible to suggest which of the many compounds may be most beneficial.

Furthermore, in the studies mentioned, controlling for other dietary variables and confounding risk factors was a difficult methodologic problem. Additional studies are needed to address the relationship of dietary-intake estimates and serum levels of the separate carotenoid components. Smoking has been associated with reductions in both dietary intake and serum levels of carotenoids, a factor that has not been adequately controlled in many analyses. Despite these many problems, prospective and retrospective nutritional (serum and dietary) epidemiologic studies, together with laboratory research, have provided important clues to the development and prevention of specific cancers. Several large-scale clinical chemoprevention trials, fueled by these data, have been initiated to investigate the protective role of β-carotene, vitamin A, or both, in epithelial neoplasia.

INTERMEDIATE–END POINT BIOMARKER STUDIES

A major goal of current basic and clinical cancer research is the identification of stage-specific biomarkers of carcinogenesis. Following initiation of carcinogenesis (genetic damage) and during the progression to invasive malignancy, epithelial cells undergo multiple (cumulative), genetically based changes associated phenotypically with dysregulated growth and differentiation. Intermediate–end point biomarkers can be defined as measurable markers of cellular and molecular events that are associated with the specific stages within the multistep evolution and progression of carcinogenesis. This definition implies that risk of cellular and molecular transformation correlates directly with the quantitative degree and pattern of biomarker expression.

Preclinical and clinical intermediate-end point studies are a rapidly growing aspect of clinical chemoprevention trials (15). These studies may require the identification of new markers that reveal earlier carcinogenic changes and a better understanding of the risk of transformation. Rapid advances in the development of microassay techniques and analysis systems have made quantitative marker measurements possible on serial sections of tiny tissue samples, a step that is a prerequisite for the integration of marker assessments into clinical chemoprevention trials. The current goal is to use these techniques to study carcinogenesis in vivo and to determine intermediate-end point markers for the cellular and molecular effects of chemopreventive agents. Although it is beyond the scope of this paper to review the status of this new and complex area of chemoprevention research (15), we wanted to familiarize the reader with its rationale before proceeding to the details of the preclinical and clinical studies that incorporate it.

PRECLINICAL STUDIES

In vitro and animal in vivo studies are invaluable for understanding the cellular and molecular evolution of epithelial carcinogenesis, establishing intermediate–end point biomarkers, screening candidate chemopreventive agents and combinations, and performing dose-response studies. Preclinical studies are fundamental to our multidisciplinary chemoprevention program at The University of Texas M. D. Anderson Cancer Center (Houston, TX).

In Vitro Studies

Our group and others are attempting to establish, maintain, and characterize human and animal cell cultures and cell lines derived from normal, premalignant, and malignant tissues with the specific goal of carcinogenesis modulation by potential chemopreventive agents. Because several of the most promising chemopreventive agents under investigation in head and neck cancer have antipromoter activity (e.g., the retinoids), the establishment of premalignant cell cultures or lines from oral mucosa would clearly be advantageous for evaluating their activities and mechanisms of action. Studies using mixed cell cultures established from biopsies of premalignant lesions, however, may be difficult to characterize and interpret. Another potential problem is that premalignant cells may continue to progress or drift toward fully transformed malignant cells in culture. This area of study is currently under intensive investigation.

In Vivo Studies

Animal models have been crucial in the study of dietary inhibitors of carcinogenesis. The hamster buccal and lingual cancer models are the most extensively studied systems in carcinogenesis and chemoprevention in the head and neck area. These and other currently available animal models use experimental carcinogens (e.g., 7,12-dimethylbenz[a]anthracene [DMBA]); unfortunately, there are no good tobacco- or alcohol-related oral cancer animal models. The evolving experimental oral SCC appears to be similar to that of the human system with respect to clinical, histologic, metabolic, biochemical, and molecular (e.g., c-erb-B) alterations (16). These models have already allowed the identification of several promising chemopreventive agents against oral carcinogenesis, including retinoic acid, β-carotene, vitamin E, selenium, and prostaglandin and protease inhibitors (16,17). Retinoic acid, for example, is highly effective in both the buccal and lingual SCC model systems, while β-carotene has chemopreventive activity in the buccal model only. Chemoprevention strategies using combinations of inhibitors based on these in vivo studies (e.g., β-carotene + α-tocopherol in buccal carcinogenesis) have led to the recent design of clinical trials.

VITAMIN A, OTHER RETINOIDS, AND CAROTENOIDS

Because of the fact that retinoids are considered prototypical differentiation agents, and both retinoids and carotenoids are used widely in the majority of both preclinical and clinical studies, a discussion of their background and potential mechanisms of action is warranted. The essential fat-soluble nutrient vitamin A, first recognized in eggs, milk, butter, and fish, is not synthesized by plants. The term "vitamin A (retinol)" now includes those substances that can restore full growth in experimental animals maintained on a vitamin A-deficient diet. The parent substance is called trans-vitamin A alcohol or trans-retinol. Its naturally occurring oxidation products are trans-retinol (vitamin A aldehyde) and trans-retinoic acid (vitamin A acid, or tretinoin). As a class of agents, these metabolites and the many synthetic analogues of vitamin A are collectively termed retinoids (14).

Carotenoids are a class of over 500 yellow- to red-hued substances chemically related to vitamin A. Found mostly in green and yellow vegetables, they also occur in tomatoes, carrots, and egg yolks. In recent years, a few carotenoids—most notably β-carotene, a dimer that is metabolized into two retinol molecules—have been studied in epidemiologic, preclinical, and early clinical studies as potential dietary inhibitors of carcinogenesis (10,11).

Mechanism of Action

A major physiologic role of vitamin A is to control cell differentiation. Preclinical studies suggest that vitamin A specifically inhibits the development of squamous epithelial carcinogenesis. Retinoids in general are potent inhibitors of the promotion phase of epithelial carcinogenesis, and suppress progression of preneoplastic lesions to invasive SCC (16). These effects may be due to inhibition of premalignant cell proliferation or to redirecting the aberrant differentiation of premalignant cells to a normal development. In fact, retinoids are established modulators of epithelial cell differentiation in vitro and in vivo. In addition, they have many other actions potentially important in their anticarcinogenic effects, including inhibition of viral (e.g., human papillomavirus) replication.

One of the major physiologic functions of vitamin A is to prevent squamous differentiation of epithelial cells in nonkeratinizing tissues (16,17). Human oral epithelium is made up of stratified squamous cells. The oral cavity mucosa is normally noncornified, except for the gingival mucosa and the mucosa on the dorsal surface of the tongue, both of which undergo keratinization. Although the mechanism or mechanisms by which retinoids prevent differentiation of squamous cells are not known, it is thought that retinoids act primarily by regulating gene expression via nuclear receptors (18). Three human nuclear retinoic acid-receptor genes that bear strong sequence homology to the presumed DNA-binding region of the member of the steroid-thyroid hormone-receptor family have been cloned (α, β, and γ).

The mechanism by which carotenoids inhibit carcinogenesis is also unclear. What is known is that the conjugated double-bond structure of carotenoids acts as a trap for singlet oxygen generated during photosynthesis, when light energy enters and is trapped by the cell. Singlet oxygen damages cellular DNA by the generation of free radicals. Therefore, carotenoids may protect cells through this mechanism by preventing cellular DNA damage. Human studies suggesting similar mechanisms have led to several chemoprevention trials for skin cancer (11). Some investigators have observed augmented tumor immunity with β-carotene in rodent models (19). A recent in vitro study of a human neuroblastoma cell line found that carotenoids suppressed proliferation and N-*myc* expression (20). In that study, α-carotene was far more active than β-carotene; this result again underscores the problem with the "positive" dietary β-carotene epidemiologic studies: they cannot possibly distinguish which of the more than 500 dietary carotenoids may be protective. Other data suggest that β-carotene's anticarcinogenic potential relates to its metabolic conversion to retinol and retinoic acid (21). The metabolic interrelationship of β-carotene and retinol has intensified the long-standing controversies regarding β-carotene's intrinsic activity and mechanism of action.

CLINICAL STUDIES

Oral Premalignancy Trials

For clinical trial design, we use the term oral premalignancy to encompass the spectrum of red, white, and speckled clinical oral lesions that cannot be scraped off or attributed to other specific disease entities, and we further classify and stratify lesions by histology as hyperplasia or mild, moderate, or severe dysplasia. Studies of the natural history of these lesions underscore two issues critical to oral chemoprevention trials: (a) all clinical premalignant lesions must be evaluated histologically; (b) to establish drug activity, randomized trials stratified by histology are required to control for the variability of the natural history.

The major demographic and etiologic factors in oral premalignancy are similar to those for oral SCC. Smoking patterns appear to influence marginally the natural history of oral premalignant lesions. Standard management, after clinical and histologic assessment, is either close observation and follow-up or surgical excision. However, excision is not feasible when there is extensive involvement; furthermore, local therapy does not prevent recurrence or multifocal development of de novo lesions. A significant number of patients, therefore, would benefit from effective chemoprevention.

Oral Leukoplakia Trials with Retinol and β-Carotene

Largely on the basis of epidemiologic and toxicity studies, several intervention studies with β-carotene have been conducted in patients with oral leukoplakia. Although establishing the safety of chemopreventive agents is very important, efficacy rates of β-carotene alone and even in combination with retinol are conflicting. Stich et al. conducted a series of trials in betel nut chewers from India using vitamin A and β-carotene alone and in combination. In one trial, Stich treated a total of 119 leukoplakia patients with either β-carotene at 180 mg/week (Group 1), β-carotene at 180 mg/week plus vitamin A at 100,000 IU/week (Group 2), or a placebo for 6 months (Group 3) (22). After the 6 months, complete remission of leukoplakia was observed in 15% of the patients in Group 1, 27% in Group 2, and 3% in Group 3. In another trial by Stich, subjects were randomly divided into two groups to receive vitamin A at 200,000 IU/week or a placebo for 6 months (23). A 57% complete remission rate was observed in the vitamin A group, with total suppression of the development of new leukoplakias. In contrast, the complete remission rate was only 3% and the new-lesion rate was 21% with placebo.

In a pilot study conducted by Garewal et al. (24), a response rate of 82% (12% complete, 70% partial response) was observed in 17 patients with oral leukoplakia who were treated with β-carotene at a dose of 30 mg/day for 3 months. In the most recently reported oral leukoplakia trial, conducted by Toma et al. (25), a response rate of only 27% was observed in 15 patients who were treated with high-dose β-carotene (90 mg/day) for 6 months. Unfortunately, none of the β-carotene studies were randomized, and in none were pretherapy and post-therapy biopsies performed to evaluate histologic response. The discrepancies in results may relate in part to the study of patient populations of differing physiologic vitamin A and β-carotene status. Results with micronutrient supplementation in vitamin A–deficient populations may be different from those of U.S. studies of pharmacologic dosing in vitamin A–replete patients.

M. D. Anderson Cancer Center Chemoprevention Trials

Our upper aerodigestive tract chemoprevention program began in 1982 with the study of the synthetic retinoid 13-*cis*–retinoic acid (13cRA). 13cRA has been extensively studied in premalignant oral lesions (26). Our rationale for using 13cRA in human premalignant oral lesions derived from pilot data using different retinoids, all given at different doses (0.5–2 mg/kg/day) and achieving response rates of 60–80% (14,26). We conducted the first controlled, double-blind, randomized trial of 13cRA versus placebo in the treatment of oral leukoplakia and reported the significant activity of high-dose (1–2 mg/kg/day) 13cRA against leukoplakia, with a clinical response rate of 67% and reversal of dysplasia in 57% after 3 months of treatment (27). In our study, there was no significant difference in responses between the patients treated with 1 mg/kg/day and those receiving 2 mg/kg/day. Toxicity at the doses used was high, even in this short-term trial. Furthermore, the relapse rate was high (>50%) within 3 months of stopping therapy.

On the basis of the results of our first trial, we developed and conducted a second study of 13cRA in oral leukoplakia. In the first 3 months, patients received 3 months of induction therapy with high-dose 13cRA (1.5 mg/kg/day) and were evaluated for histologic and clinical responses and biomarker changes (micronuclei and squamous-differentiation markers). Preliminary results obtained from our analyses, which indicated the feasibility and modulation of biomarkers, have been reviewed elsewhere (15). After the 3-month induction phase, patients were randomized to a 9-month treatment with either low-dose 13cRA (0.5 mg/kg/day) or β-carotene (30 mg/day). The patients selected for this study had histologically confirmed, measurable, premalignant oral lesions (either dysplastic or extensive, symptomatic, hyperplastic lesions). There was a significantly lower relapse rate with maintenance low-dose 13cRA compared with β-carotene. The data indicated that low-dose 13cRA is effective and well-tolerated maintenance therapy for oral premalignancy (28).

We have also evaluated maintenance effects on micronuclei frequency, an easily quantitated biomarker of ongoing genotoxicity. We observed a micronuclei pattern reflective of the clinical maintenance data: low-dose 13cRA more effectively maintained or further reduced micronuclei frequencies compared with β-carotene (28). Another recent study monitored micronuclei as a measure of efficacy of maintenance chemopreventive therapy; its data, consistent with our 13cRA data, indicated that retinol was more effective than β-carotene in maintaining micronuclei suppression (16).

We also conducted a prospective, randomized adjuvant chemoprevention trial of high-dose 13cRA (50–100 mg/m^2) versus placebo in head and neck SCC (29). The rationale for this already-completed study, which enrolled over 100 patients, was derived from the concept of field cancerization, the magnitude of the clinical problem of second primary tumors in head and neck cancer (4) and, regarding 13cRA itself, the promising preclinical (in vitro and in vivo) and epidemiologic data, the significant clinical activity in oral leukoplakia (27), and the activity (though modest) in advanced head and neck SCC (30).

Our analyses of the two major classes of failure patterns—(a) second primary tumors and (b) local, regional, and distant recurrences—revealed that the 13cRA treatment significantly reduced the incidence of second primary tumor development. Only two patients (4%) in the 13cRA arm developed a second primary tumor versus 12 patients (24%) in the placebo arm ($P = 0.005$ on direct comparison at a median follow-up of 32 months). Multiple second primary tumors occurred in four patients, all of whom were in the placebo group. No significant differences appeared between the two patient groups in regard to local, regional, or distant recurrences. Toxicity in the 13cRA group, consisting of mucocutaneous dryness and asymptomatic hypertriglyceridemia, was more severe and more often intolerable than in the placebo group.

Smoking is indisputably the major risk factor in the development of initial primary cancer of the upper aerodigestive tract and lung. However, the quantitative impact of smoking cessation on the development of second primaries is unclear (4,16). It appears that after definitive therapy of the primary head and neck cancer, the probability of a second primary is determined chiefly by exposures (e.g., from tobacco) received before the initial cancer was diagnosed. In our study, four of the 14 patients (29%) who developed second primary cancer were active (or current) smokers. These data underscore the need for an effective chemoprevention strategy against second primaries in head and neck cancer.

All patients in this study were followed prospectively and monitored closely at regular intervals. The resulting data gave us precise information on the patterns of second primary development. The second primary cancer was SCC occurring in the upper aerodigestive tract, esophagus, or lung in 13 of our 14 patients (93%). This pattern corresponds with the site-dispersal patterns of second primary disease reported in other head and neck cancer series (exclusive of nasopharyngeal and salivary gland cancer) and is consistent with the results predicted by tobacco-related field cancerization.

Because head and neck cancer is a significant public health problem, chemoprevention with 13cRA is attractive, but by no means has it been adequately tested. The results of our placebo-controlled, randomized trial have established the significant adjuvant activity of this agent at high doses in preventing second primary tumors in squamous cell carcinoma of the head and neck. Our toxicity data and the necessity of long-term therapy, however, suggest the need for new chemoprevention approaches to controlling head and neck cancer. Given these 13cRA data and our data showing the effectiveness and mild toxicity of low-dose 13cRA, we are preparing a trial to investigate the efficacy and safety of low-dose 13cRA for preventing second primary tumors in early-stage head and neck cancer. Furthermore, we are now expanding this line of study to early-stage, non-small cell lung cancer, with a rationale in the field cancerization concept and similar rate of second primary tumors.

TOXICITY ISSUES

Establishing the safety of chemopreventive agents for use by relatively healthy individuals at varying degrees of risk is of major importance. Short- and long-term toxicities must be carefully studied before exposing thousands of subjects for many years. The balance between efficacy and toxicity is very delicate in the area of chemoprevention and will likely vary with lesions of differing transformation risk.

β-Carotene as used thus far has had no clinical toxic effects, except for dose-dependent skin yellowing. There may be other problems with long-term β-carotene supplementation, which is just beginning to be studied. For example, β-carotene dosing at 30 mg/day (most chemoprevention trials have used 30–50 mg/day) was found to produce a highly significant decrease in plasma α-tocopherol (vitamin E) levels (31). Since α-tocopherol is a potent chemopreventive agent in hamster cheek-pouch models and is currently undergoing clinical trial (17), this effect of β-carotene could potentially be harmful, and in fact increase cancer risk.

The major drawback in the use of retinoids for chemoprevention is the associated dose-dependent, reversible, mucocutaneous toxicity, the mechanism of which is not clear. Patient compliance, limited by this toxicity, is a major problem in the design of long-term studies. Since retinoic acid derivatives (at high doses) are the only chemopreventive agents that have been proved active clinically (27,32) and may be very important in the therapy of some malignancies (30,33), there is now great interest in evaluating ways to reduce or control their toxic effects.

Three promising areas of investigation are currently under way. The first concerns identifying the lowest effective dose of 13cRA. Until now, all reported retinoid trials have empirically used more than 0.5 mg/kg/day. Since toxicity is dose related, it is important to determine the clinical, histologic, and biologic activity of lower-dose 13cRA using a systematic study design. Oral premalignancy is an ideal model system for a dose-searching study not only because of its intrinsic features (e.g., easily monitored lesions) but also because of the established activity of high-dose retinoic acid in this setting. The incorporation of more sensitive intermediate–end point biomarkers is especially appropriate for this line of work.

The second line of investigation was stimulated by a University of Pennsylvania clinical myelodysplasia study (34) in which oral α-tocopherol (800 mg/day) was found to markedly reduce the clinical and laboratory (especially lipid) toxic effects of high-dose 13cRA (100 mg/ m^2). Moreover, this drug combination was very active. The interaction between vitamin A analogues and vitamin E is not well understood. However, if it is clinically confirmed (regardless of the precise mechanistic details), this interactive effect will be a major impetus in the use of retinoids in cancer prevention and treatment.

The third line of study is the synthesis and screening of newer, less toxic retinoids, such as retinamides (14). Promising results have been obtained in a human breast trial and an animal tracheal model trial utilizing the retinamide 4-HPR. Further study of this and other compounds is an exciting new area in the field of chemoprevention that will hopefully yield less toxic long-term treatment regimens (14).

Retinol is well tolerated within a fairly wide dose range. Doses of 200,000 IU/day produced no toxic effects (16). However, doses of 350,000–400,000 IU/day were associated with toxicity, albeit nonspecific reactions (e.g., headache and skin dryness), in one third of patients. Short-term retinoid toxic effects are dose dependent and reversible. The synthetic retinoids are comparable to vitamin A in their spectrum of toxicity. The most common toxic effects are mucocutaneous dryness (cheilitis, xerosis, photosensitivity), musculoskeletal complaints, and headache. Laboratory abnormalities include asymptomatic increases in serum triglycerides (30–40%) and aminotransferases (10–15%). Subclinical ocular toxic effects may be associated with all synthetic retinoids, although symptomatic night blindness is uncommon (35).

The most serious potential problem of treatment with retinoids is the severe teratogenic effects reported in infants exposed in utero. Therefore, women of childbearing potential must be excluded from retinoid chemoprevention trials. In chemoprevention trials of tobacco-related epithelial neoplasia, however, this issue pertains to only a small minority of subjects. Bone toxicity (i.e., premature epiphyseal closure) is a particular concern in pediatric patients receiving prolonged high-dose 13cRA therapy for hyperkeratotic skin disorders. In adults, the majority develop asymptomatic extraspinal tendon and ligament calcification (14).

Other promising chemopreventive agents have not been well studied for toxicity in clinical trials. The National Cancer Institute, however, has recently begun formal Phase I testing of several new drugs (17). However, evaluation for their chronic side effects, the primary toxicity issue for chemopreventive drugs, will take many years.

CONCLUSIONS

Although tobacco-related aerodigestive tract neoplasms are a major, increasing worldwide problem, chemoprevention offers a promising new approach to its control. Head and neck cancer is an excellent model for the study of epithelial carcinogenesis and its chemoprevention. Lessons learned from the pioneering work in this cancer system may now be extended to other epithelial cancers, such as lung and esophageal cancers. For example, clinical trial design issues, including the great importance of randomized, placebo-controlled trials to establish drug efficacy in premalignancy, are critical in light of the variable natural history of oral and other epithelial premalignant lesions.

The preclinical in vitro and animal studies in head and neck carcinogenesis are also generating a wealth of information concerning the potential application of chemopreventive agents. As with the clinical trials, these studies require well-controlled, focused designs addressing specific issues. The results from specific preclinical and clinical studies, however, may not apply to other settings, even with only slightly modified designs within the same carcinogenesis system.

High-dose 13cRA is the only chemopreventive agent that has been proved effective in humans. The systematic study and development of this drug have set the stage for the similar study of new drugs. Studies using buccal and lingual carcinogenesis models, the best head and neck cancer models, have strongly supported the chemopreventive role of retinoids. Results from these positive, nonrandomized clinical retinoid trials in oral premalignancy were confirmed by a randomized high-dose 13cRA study. These retinoid oral premalignancy studies in turn presaged the efficacy of high-dose 13cRA in significantly preventing second primary tumors in a randomized trial in head and neck cancer patients. In fact, promising data on lower-dose 13cRA in human oral premalignancies have now led to the design of large-scale studies of this less toxic approach in the prevention of second primary tumors in head and neck and lung cancers.

A major issue in all forms of cancer control, the fine balance between toxicity and efficacy (and cancer risk), is an even greater concern in chemopreventive efforts in relatively healthy subjects. Patients with acute promyelocytic leukemia are less likely to be concerned about retinoid-related skin dryness than are healthy, albeit high-risk, subjects. Some chemotherapeutic agents, such as supplemental β-carotene, cause little or no clinical side effects, but concern is growing about their administration because of hidden toxicities, such as detrimental interactions with α-tocopherol and, possibly, other critical micronutrients.

In a field in which only one agent has proven activity, the efficacy issue is critical. This important perspective suggests that it is equally as important (if not more so) to investigate better, less toxic ways to use proven drugs as to develop new, currently unproven agents. Twenty years ago, cisplatin was shelved because of its high toxicity; now, as its toxicity has been addressed and ways to control its toxicity have been found, this drug is one of the best antineoplastics there is. Skin dryness from 13cRA, although obviously far less severe than standard chemotherapy toxic effects, is still of some concern with high doses, especially for long-term use. Studies of ways to reduce this agent's toxicity are under way and include systematic studies of lower doses, trials of new (less toxic) synthetic analogues, and studies to confirm the ameliorating activity seen in α-tocopherol.

β-Carotene, very attractive from a toxicity perspective, is unproven as a chemopreventive agent. Response rates in oral premalignancy studies are conflicting, with high-dose, long-term protocols producing low response rates (<30%), roughly in the range of spontaneous change rates, and with one uncontrolled clinical study showing an overall response rate of 82% with lower-dose, short-term therapy. Uncontrolled pilot studies in this area of investigation are misleading and dangerous to the general public in many regards, not the least of which is the false sense of security given to high-risk subjects, who may take β-carotene *and* continue to smoke. Controlled, randomized trials are critical in situations such as this.

Because epithelial cancers develop during a prolonged, multistep process that may last decades, chemoprevention trials that are conducted in high-risk subjects and that use incidence of invasive cancer as the end point have serious feasibility problems. To establish efficacy, these trials require the study of thousands of subjects for 5–10 years (or longer) and at greater cost than with standard chemotherapy trials. Short-term, in vivo, intermediate–end point biomarkers, often identified in preclinical studies, will probably play an increasingly important role in the design of scientifically sound chemoprevention trials by helping researchers establish optimal drugs, doses, and schedules for specific chemoprevention trials.

ACKNOWLEDGMENT

This work was supported, in part, by National Cancer Institute Grants CA-48303 and CA-48369.

REFERENCES

1. Silverberg E, Boring CC, Squires TS. Cancer statistics, 1990. CA 40:9–26, 1990.
2. Hong WK, Bromer R. Chemotherapy in head and neck cancer. N Engl J Med 308:75–79, 1983.
3. Hong WK, Bromer RH, Amato DA, Shapshay S, Vincent M, Vaughan C, Willett B, Katz A, Welch J, Fofonoff S, Strong MS. Patterns of relapse in locally advanced head and neck cancer patients who achieved complete remission after combined modality therapy. Cancer 56:1242–1245, 1985.
4. Lippman SM, Hong WK. Second malignant tumors in head and neck squamous cell carcinoma: The overshadowing threat for patients with early-stage disease (editorial). Int J Radiat Oncol Biol Phys 17:691–694, 1989.
5. Slaughter DP, Southwick HW, Smejkal W. "Field cancerization" in oral stratified squamous epithelium: Clinical implications of multicentric origin. Cancer 6:963–968, 1953.
6. Devesa SS, Silverman DT, Young JL, Pollack ES, Brown CC, Horm JW, Percy CL, Myers MH, McKay FW, Fraumeni JF Jr. Cancer incidence and mortality trends among whites in the United States. J Natl Cancer Inst 79:701–741, 1987.
7. Decker J, Goldstein JC. Risk factors in head and neck cancer. N Engl J Med 306:1151–1155, 1982.
8. Brandsma J, Abramson AL. Association of papillomavirus with cancers of the head and neck. Arch Otolaryngol Head Neck Surg 115:621–625, 1989.
9. Spitz MR, Fueger JJ, Beddingfield NA, Annegers JF, Hsu TC, Newell GR, Schantz SP. Chromosome sensitivity to bleomycin-induced mutagenesis: An independent risk factor for upper aerodigestive tract cancers. Cancer Res 49:4626–4628, 1989.
10. Peto R, Doll R, Buckley JD, Sporn MB. Can dietary beta-carotene materially reduce human cancer rates? Nature 290:201–208, 1981.
11. Bertram JS, Kolonel LN, Meyskens FL Jr. Rationale and strategies for chemoprevention of cancer in humans. Cancer Res 47:3012–3031, 1987.
12. Ziegler RG. A review of epidemiologic evidence that carotenoids reduce the risk of cancer. J Nutr 119:116–122, 1989.
13. Winn DM, Ziegler RG, Pickle LW, Gridley G, Blot WJ, Hoover RN. Diet in the etiology of oral and pharyngeal cancer among women from the southern United States. Cancer Res 44:1216–1222, 1984.
14. Lippman SM, Kessler JF, Meyskens FL Jr. Retinoids as preventive and therapeutic anticancer agents. Cancer Treatment Reports 71(4) Part I:391–405, 71(5) Part II:493–515, 1987.
15. Lippman SM, Lee JS, Lotan R, Hittelman W, Wargovich MJ, Hong WK. Biomarkers as intermediate end points in chemoprevention trials. J Natl Cancer Inst 82:550–560, 1990.
16. Lippman SM, Hong WK. Differentiation therapy for head and neck cancer. In Snow G, Clark JR (eds). Multimodality Therapy for Head and Neck Cancer. New York: Georg Thieme Verlag, in press.
17. Lippman SM, Lee JS, Lotan R, Hong WK. Chemoprevention of Upper Aerodigestive Cancer Task Force Workshop. Head Neck 12:5–20, 1990.
18. Evans RM. The steroid and thyroid hormone receptor superfamily. Science 240:889–895, 1988.
19. Tomita Y, Himeno K, Nomoto K, Endo H, Hirohata T. Augmentation of tumor immunity against syngeneic tumors in mice by beta-carotene. J Natl Cancer Inst 78:679–681, 1987.
20. Murakoshi M, Takayasu J, Kimura O, Kohmura E, Nishino H, Iwashima A, Okuzumi J, Sakai T, Sugimoto T, Imanishi J. Inhibitory effects of alpha-carotene on proliferation of the human neuroblastoma cell line GOTO. J Natl Cancer Inst 81:1649–1652, 1989.

21. Napoli JL, Race KR. Biogenesis of retinoic acid from β-carotene: Differences between the metabolism of β-carotene and retinol. J Biol Chem 263:17372–17377, 1988.
22. Stich HF, Rosin MP, Hornby AP, Mathew B, Sankaranarayanan R, Nair MK. Remission of oral leukoplakias and micronuclei in tobacco/betel quid chewers treated with beta-carotene and with beta-carotene plus vitamin A. Int J Cancer 42:195–199, 1988.
23. Stich HF, Hornby AP, Mathew B, Sankaranarayanan R, Nair MK. Response of oral leukoplakias to the administration of vitamin A. Cancer Lett 40:93–101, 1988.
24. Garewal H, Allen V, Killen D, Elletson H, Reeves D, King D, Meyskens F. Beta-carotene (BC) is an effective, non-toxic agent for the treatment of premalignant lesions of the oral cavity (abstract). Proceedings of the American Society of Clinical Oncology Annual Meeting 8:167, 1989.
25. Toma S, Albanese E, De Lorenzi M, Nicolo G, Mangiante P, Galli A, Cancedda R. Beta-carotene in the treatment of oral leukoplakia (abstract). Proceedings of the Annual Meeting of the American Society of Clinical Oncology 9:179, 1990.
26. Lippman SM, Garewal HS, Meyskens FL Jr. Retinoids as potential chemopreventive agents in squamous cell carcinoma of the head and neck. Prev Med 18:740–748, 1989.
27. Hong WK, Endicott J, Itri LM, Doos W, Batsakis JG, Bell R, Fofonoff S, Byers R, Atkinson EN, Vaughan C, Toth BB, Kramer A, Dimery IW, Skipper P, Strong S. 13-cis-Retinoic acid in the treatment of oral leukoplakia. N Engl J Med 315:1501–1505, 1986.
28. Lippman SM, Toth BB, Batsakis JG, Lee JS, Weber RS, McCarthy KS, Martin JW, Hay SG, Wargovich MJ, Lotan R, Hong WK. Low-dose 13-cis-retinoic acid (13cRA) maintains remission in oral premalignancy: More effective than β-carotene in randomized trial (abstract). Proceedings of the Annual Meeting of the American Society of Clinical Oncology 9:225, 1990.
29. Hong WK, Lippman SM, Itri LM, Karp DD, Lee JS, Byers RM, Schantz SP, Kramer AM, Lotan R, Peters LJ, Dimery IW, Brown BW, Goepfert H. Prevention of second primary tumors in squamous cell carcinoma of the head and neck with 13-cis-retinoic acid. N Engl J Med 323:795–800, 1990.
30. Lippman SM, Kessler JF, Al-Sarraf M, Alberts DS, Itri LM, Mattox D, Von Hoff DD, Loescher L, Meyskens FL. Treatment of advanced squamous cell carcinoma of the head and neck with isotretinoin: A phase II randomized trial. Invest New Drugs 6:51–56, 1988.
31. Xu MJ, Pneg UM, Liu Y, Alberts DS, Plezla PM, Sayers SM. Effect of chronic oral administration of β-carotene on plasma α-tocopherol concentrations in normal subjects (abstract). Proceedings of the American Association for Cancer Research 31:126, 1990.
32. Kraemer KH, DiGiovanna JJ, Moshell AN, Tarone RE, Peck GL. Prevention of skin cancer in xeroderma pigmentosum with the use of oral isotretinoin. N Engl J Med 318:1633–1637, 1988.
33. Lippman SM, Meyskens FL Jr. Treatment of advanced squamous cell carcinoma of the skin with isotretinoin. Ann Intern Med 107:499–502, 1987.
34. Besa EC, Abrahm JL, Nowell PC. Comparison of efficacy and toxicity of 13-cis-retinoic acid (RA) with or without alpha tocopherol in myelodysplasia (abstract). Proceedings of the American Society of Hematology 70:222a, 1987.
35. Modiano MR, Dalton WS, Lippman SM, Joffe L, Booth AR, Meyskens FL Jr. Ocular toxic effects of fenretinide. J Natl Cancer Inst 82:1063, 1990.

CONTRIBUTORS

Ingalill Avis
National Cancer Institute
U.S. PHS, Bldg. 8, Rm. 5101
NNMC 8901 Wisconsin Avenue
Bethesda, Maryland 20814-5101

Michael Birrer
National Cancer Institute
U.S. PHS, Bldg. 8, Rm. 5101
NNMC 8901 Wisconsin Avenue
Bethesda, Maryland 20814-5101

Robert M. Byers
Department of Head and Neck Surgery, Box 69
The University of Texas M. D. Anderson
    Cancer Center
1515 Holcombe Boulevard
Houston, Texas 77030

Thomas E. Carey
Department of Otolaryngology, Head and Neck
    Surgery
University of Michigan Cancer Center
Ann Arbor, Michigan 48109

Frank Cuttitta
National Cancer Institute
U.S. PHS, Bldg. 8, Rm. 5101
NNMC 8901 Wisconsin Avenue
Bethesda, Maryland 20814-5101

Dennis L. Cooper
Department of Medical Oncology
Yale University School of Medicine
26 High Street
New Haven, Connecticut 06510

Carol J. Detrisac
Life Sciences Research
IIT Research Institute
10 West 35th Street
Chicago, Illinois 60616

Barbara G. Fallon
Section of Hematology/Oncology
St. Francis Hospital and Medical Center
114 Woodland Street
Hartford, Connecticut 06105-1299

Craig D. Friedman
Department of Surgery
Yale University School of Medicine
26 High Street
New Haven, Connecticut 06510

Harinder S. Garewal
Section of Hematology and Oncology
Tucson VA Medical Center
Tucson, Arizona 85723

Irma B. Gimenez-Conti
The University of Texas M. D. Anderson
    Cancer Center
Science Park—Research Division
P.O. Box 389
Smithville, Texas 78957

Gary E. Goodman
Swedish Hospital Medical Center Tumor
    Institute
Seattle, Washington 98104

W. Jarrard Goodwin, Jr.
Department of Otolaryngology
University of Miami School of Medicine
Miami, Florida 33124

Waun Ki Hong
Section of Head, Neck, and Thoracic Medical
    Oncology, Box 80
The University of Texas M. D. Anderson
    Cancer Center
1515 Holcombe Boulevard
Houston, Texas 77030

T.C. Hsu
Department of Cell Biology, Box 181
The University of Texas M. D. Anderson
Cancer Center
1515 Holcombe Boulevard
Houston, Texas 77030

Dwight T. Janerich
Cancer Prevention Research Unit for
Connecticut at Yale
Yale University School of Medicine
26 High Street
New Haven, Connecticut 06510

Anton M. Jetten
National Institutes of Health
Environmental Health Sciences
P.O. Box 12233
Research Triangle Park, North Carolina 27709

Gary J. Kelloff
Chemoprevention Branch
National Cancer Institute
Bethesda, Maryland 20892

Leena Laurikainen
Department of Otolaryngology, Head and Neck
Surgery
University of Michigan Cancer Center
Ann Arbor, Michigan 48109

Keith Linder
Department of Otolaryngology, Head and Neck
Surgery
University of Michigan Cancer Center
Ann Arbor, Michigan 48109

Scott M. Lippman
Department of Medical Oncology, Box 80
The University of Texas M. D. Anderson
Cancer Center
1515 Holcombe Boulevard
Houston, Texas 77030

Cynthia Marcelo
Department of Dermatology
University of Michigan Cancer Center
Ann Arbor, Michigan 48109

Susan Taylor Mayne
Cancer Prevention Research Unit for
Connecticut at Yale
Yale University School of Medicine
26 High Street
New Haven, Connecticut 06510

Jerry W. McLarty
Epidemiology/Biomathematics
The University of Texas Health Science Center
at Tyler
P.O. Box 2003
Tyler, Texas 75710

Curtis J. Mettlin
Department of Cancer Prevention and
Epidemiology
Roswell Park Cancer Institute
666 Elm Street
Buffalo, New York 14263

Richard C. Moon
Life Sciences Research
IIT Research Institute
10 West 35th Street
Chicago, Illinois 60616

Thomas E. Moon
Department of Family and Community
Medicine
University of Arizona Cancer Center
Tucson, Arizona 85724

James L. Mulshine
National Cancer Institute
U.S. PHS, Bldg. 8, Rm. 5101
NNMC 8901 Wisconsin Avenue
Bethesda, Maryland 20814-5101

Thankam S. Nair
Department of Otolaryngology, Head and Neck
Surgery
University of Michigan Cancer Center
Ann Arbor, Michigan 48109

Guy R. Newell
Department of Cancer Prevention and Control,
Box 189
The University of Texas M. D. Anderson
Cancer Center
1515 Holcombe Boulevard
Houston, Texas 77030

Clara Nervi
National Institutes of Health
Environmental Health Sciences
P.O. Box 12233
Research Triangle Park, North Carolina 27709

Gilbert S. Omenn
*Swedish Hospital Medical Center Tumor
    Institute
Seattle, Washington 98104*

Angelika Ptok
*Department of Otolaryngology, Head and Neck
    Surgery
University of Michigan Cancer Center
Ann Arbor, Michigan 48109*

Kathryn Quinn
*National Cancer Institute
U.S. PHS, Bldg. 8, Rm. 5101
NNMC 8901 Wisconsin Avenue
Bethesda, Maryland 20814-5101*

Kandala V.N. Rao
*Life Sciences Research
IIT Research Institute
10 West 35th Street
Chicago, Illinois 60616*

Barbara K. Rimer
*Cancer Control Research Program
Duke Comprehensive Cancer Center, Box 2949
Duke University Medical Center
Durham, North Carolina 27710*

Timothy Reinke
*Department of Otolaryngology, Head and Neck
    Surgery
University of Michigan Cancer Center
Ann Arbor, Michigan 48109*

Miriam P. Rosin
*Division of Epidemiology, Biometry and
    Occupational Oncology
Cancer Control Agency of British Columbia
600 West 10th Avenue
Vancouver, British Columbia, V5Z 4E6,
    CANADA*

Stimson P. Schantz
*Department of Head and Neck Surgery
Memorial Sloan-Kettering Cancer Center
New York, New York 10021*

David Schottenfeld
*University of Michigan School of Public Health
109 Observatory Street
Ann Arbor, Michigan 48109-2029*

Frank Scott
*National Institutes of Health
Environmental Health Sciences
P.O. Box 12233
Research Triangle Park, North Carolina 27709*

Margaret R. Spitz
*Department of Cancer Prevention
    and Control, Box 189
The University of Texas M. D. Anderson
    Cancer Center
1515 Holcombe Boulevard
Houston, Texas 77030*

Thomas J. Slaga
*The University of Texas M. D. Anderson
    Cancer Center
Science Park—Research Division
P.O. Box 389
Smithville, Texas 78957*

Anthony M. Treston
*National Cancer Institute
U.S. PHS, Bldg. 8, Rm. 5101
NNMC 8901 Wisconsin Avenue
Bethesda, Maryland 20814-5101*

Bruce Trock
*Division of Population Science
Fox Chase Cancer Center
510 Township Line Road
Cheltenham, Pennsylvania 19012*

Thomas M. Vollberg
*National Institutes of Health
Environmental Health Sciences
P.O. Box 12233
Research Triangle Park, North Carolina 27709*

Deborah M. Winn
*Division of Health Interviews Statistics
National Center for Health Statistics
3700 East West Highway
Hyattsville, Maryland 20782*

Tongzhang Zheng
*Cancer Prevention Research Unit for
    Connecticut at Yale
Yale University School of Medicine
26 High Street
New Haven, Connecticut 06510*

INDEX

Hamster
  buccal and lingual cancer models, 154
  buccal pouch model and β-carotene,
    120–121
  cheek pouch model, 63–66, 132
  lung cancer model, 55–59
Head and neck cancer; *see* Cancer, head and
    neck
Hemoglobin adducts, 43–44
Her-2/neu gene, 85–86
Herpes virus, 42, 152
Hyaluronidase synthesis, 91
4-Hydroxyphenyl-retinamide, 58, 131
Hyperplasia, 65–66, 89–90, 91
Hypervitaminosis, 142

Infection, 98–99
Inflammation, 98–99
Insulin-like growth factor I, 82, 89–90
Intervention
  adherence to, 107–108, 113–115
  dietary vs. pharmacologic, 25
  simultaneous testing of multiple, 106

Keratin, 63–64, 65, 91
Keratinocyte growth factor, 89–90

Laryngeal cancer; *see* Cancer, laryngeal
Lesions, premalignant, 129
Leukoplakia, *see* Oral leukoplakia
Lung cancer; *see* Cancer, lung
Lymphoepithelial carcinoma, 6

Markers, biologic, 43 (*see also* Micronu-
    clei)
  definition and applications, 47, 153
  in detection, 85
  panels of, 53
  that predict prognosis, 48–51
  and response to therapy, 51–53
  sensitivity and specificity, 48
  usefulness criteria, 47–48
Markers, genetic, 34, 86
Mesothelioma, 141
Metaplasia, premalignant, 130
Methylguanine, 43
4-(*N*-methyl-*N*-nitrosamino)-1-(3-pyridyl)-
    1-butanone (NNK), 40, 43
N-methyl-*N*-nitrosourea, 55–56
Micronuclei (*see also* Markers, biologic)
  and clinical maintenance data, 156
  during carcinogenesis, 65

Micronuclei (continued)
  evaluating efficacy of chemopreventives,
    99–102, 121, 132
  formation of, 95
  and genetic changes, 97
  and oral cancer, 132
  in screening, 53, 96
  in smokeless tobacco users, 44
Monoclonal antibody
  anti-GRP, 82
  UM-A9, 70
Mouse skin model of carcinogenesis, 63
Mucosa, oral cavity, 154
Mutagen sensitivity, 32–35

Nasopharyngeal carcinoma, 6–8
Nitrosamines, 40, 43
N-nitrosodimethylamine, 12, 57
N-nitrosonornicotine, 40, 43
Nucleolar organizer regions, 65
Nutrition, *see* Diet

Oral cancer; *see* Cancer, oral
Oral leukoplakia
  and β-carotene, 121, 133, 142, 143, 155
  chemopreventive goals, 132
  and 13cRA, 132–133, 156–157
  clinical response criteria, 133
  definition, 131
  in hamster cheek pouch model, 65
  micronuclei test in, 101–102
  and retinol, 155
  in smokeless tobacco users, 41–42
  treatment of, 132–133
  and vitamin A, 132–133
Ornithine decarboxylase, 65, 130

p53 gene, 85–86
p62 protein, 51
Pan, 42, 152
Papillomavirus, 152
Pharyngeal cancer; *see* Cancer, pharyngeal
Phenotype, squamous-differentiated, 91
Phosphohexose isomerase, 52
Pipe smoking, 10 (*see also* Tobacco)
Pleural disease, nonmalignant, 141
Polonium 210, 40
Polyamine, 65, 130
Praziquantel, 99
Premalignancy
  lesions, 129
  oral, 155, 158

Prevention, *see* Chemoprevention
Prostaglandin inhibitor, 154
Protease inhibitor, 154
Proteins, retinoic acid–binding, 92
Putrescine, 65

Radiation
  and development of SCC, 152
  and second cancer, 27
Rapid Case Ascertainment system, 122
ras gene, 85–86
Relationship, participant-researcher,
        113–114
Retinamides, 158
Retinoic acid, 154
Retinoic acid–binding proteins, cytosolic,
        92
Retinoic acid receptors, 92
Retinoids, 138 (*see also* 13-*cis*-retinoic
        acid)
  animal studies in prevention, 137–138
  antitumor properties, 142
  chemopreventive trials of, 138–140
  effectiveness, 59
  and gene expression, 92
  history of use, 57–58
  in utero effects, 158
  and leukoplakia, 132–134
  mechanism of action, 92, 154–155
  role in cell growth/differentiation, 91–93
  toxicity, 158
Retinol, 58, 141–143
  animal studies, 137–138
  as a cancer risk, 123
  clinical trial in asbestos workers,
        143–147
  efficacy, 155
  toxicity, 158
Retinyl acetate, 58
Retinyl palmitate, 58
  chemoprevention trial, 100–101, 138–139
  and lung cancer relapse, 81
Reverse chutta, 152
Run-in period, 108, 113, 123

Schistosoma, 98–99
Scotch whiskey, 35
Second primary tumors; *see* Cancer, second
        primary
Selenium, 58, 154
Sialic acid, 52

Snuff, 10 (*see also* Tobacco, smokeless)
  and cancer, 11, 39–42, 44
  history of use, 39–40
  micronuclei test in users, 101
Spermidine, 65
Spermine, 65
Sputum
  atypia, 146, 147
  cytology, 84–85, 143
  squamous metaplasia, 143
Squamous carcinoma
  morbidity, 119
  multiple primary, 27–30
Stability, genomic, 96
Superoxidase dismutase, 97

Tamoxifen, 83
Tax, California cigarette, 81
12-*O*-tetradecanoylphorbol-13-acetate,
        65–66
Tissue trauma, 98
Tobacco (*see also* Cigar smoking; Cigarette
        smoking; Pipe smoking; Snuff;
        Tobacco, smokeless; Tobacco,
        chewing)
  advertising, 40
  and alcohol, 13, 36
  brands, 43
  carcinogens in, 9
  chemical analysis of, 10
  composition, 9
  curing, 10
  and esophageal cancer, 14
  and laryngeal cancer, 12, 14
  and oral cancer, 2, 12, 14, 40–41, 132,
        152
  and second cancer, 28–29
  use statistics, 151
Tobacco, chewing, 10 (*see also* Tobacco,
        smokeless)
  additives in, 11
  and aerodigestive tract cancer, 39–42, 44
  demographics, 11
  history of use, 39
Tobacco, smokeless, 40–44 (*see also*
        Tobacco, chewing and Snuff)
α-tocopherol, 158
Toxicity
  of β-carotene, 124–125, 142, 147,
        157–158
  of chemopreventive agents, 134, 159
  of 13-*cis*–retinoic acid, 135, 156, 157